STUBBORN
GRACE

STUBBORN GRACE

FAITH, MENTAL ILLNESS, & DEMANDING A BLESSING

Kate Landis

Skinner House Books

Boston

www.skinnerhouse.org
Printed in the United States

Cover design by Kathryn Sky-Peck
Text design by Jeff Miller
Author photo by Dane Scott

print ISBN: 978-1-55896-857-8
eBook ISBN: 978-1-55896-858-5

6 5 4 3 2 1
23 22 21 20

Library of Congress Cataloging-in-Publication Data
Names: Landis, Kate, author.
Title: Stubborn grace : faith, mental illness, and demanding a blessing : a memoir / by Kate Landis.
Description: Boston : Skinner House Books, [2020]
Identifiers: LCCN 2020018624 (print) | LCCN 2020018625 (ebook) | ISBN 9781558968578 (paperback) | ISBN 9781558968585 (ebook)
Subjects: LCSH: Landis, Kate. | Unitarian Universalist Association—Clergy—Biography.
Classification: LCC BX9869.L36 A3 2020 (print) | LCC BX9869.L36 (ebook) | DDC 289.1092 [B]—dc23
LC record available at https://lccn.loc.gov/2020018624
LC ebook record available at https://lccn.loc.gov/2020018625

For Jay,

*All the hair band lyrics of the 1980s
cannot express how much
I love you.*

Contents

Introduction ix

1. The Incomplete Castle 1
2. The Family Curse 4
3. Emma and Wilma 12
4. It's All Jimmy Carter's Fault 20
5. Choose Jesus . . . or Else 30
6. Sadness the Chimp and the Evil Katieo 37
7. Mad Dog the Angry Adolescent 50
8. Technicolor Romance 68
9. Psych Hospital, Version One 80
10. Off the Roof 99
11. Electric Hallelujah 103
12. Sharon Jumped 114
13. No Resurrection for Cool Girls 127
14. Great Jobs I Got Fired From 137
15. The Patriarchy Always Knocks Twice 152

16. Good Choices, Bad Reasons 162

17. Stealing Junk 165

18. Accidentally Stealing 170

19. Two Pink Lines 179

20. Big Sister God 191

21. Starting Single 210

22. Once Burned, Twice Shy 216

23. Fasten Your Theological Seatbelt 221

24. Like in Washington? 227

25. The Dalai Lama Says I'm Okay.
My Niece Disagrees. 231

26. Refusing to Be Enemies 240

27. A Streetcar Named Dignity 249

28. Good Guys 256

29. Ferocious Love 262

30. Heaven Is a Place on Earth 269

31. Riding Horses to Heaven 277

32. Spiritual Safety Rails 286

33. But You'll Die! 297

34. Jazz Hands for the Prodigal Son 305

Benediction 313

Introduction

IT IS SUNDAY MORNING and I'm swearing at my alarm—
there is no way it's morning, I went to bed ten minutes
ago.... But weak sunlight is angling around the curtain
and into my room, so yes, morning has arrived. Running
my hands through my pink hair, smoothing the spikes into
the semblance of curls, I gobble a peanut butter sandwich
on my way out the door. The cool morning air clears my
mental spiderwebs, and I'm off to church.

Around me the city lies silent. The roads are empty,
except for annoyingly perky joggers in reflective vests and
toddlers being chased by sleepy parents. My friends will not
wake for hours, and even then, brunch will be their first
priority, not getting to Sunday morning worship service. Is
it possible that the most countercultural thing about me
is that I go to church? Sure, I have pink hair, and sure, I
danced all night to a raucous feminist punk band, but my

participation in a faith community is what sets me apart from my peers. Why do I press myself out of bed at this ungodly hour (pun intended) to sit in a room with a bunch of other people and sing songs, light candles, and meditate?

I live in one of the most secular parts of the US, and I'm a part of that small movement of young people who go to church not because it would be socially weird not to, but because we are looking for greater depth in our lives. This isn't the Deep South—nearly all of the people going to church in Seattle are fundamentalists. When I tell people at concerts or parties that I am a minister, they back away slowly, and when I explain my liberal faith, they think it's cute in a twee, old-timey way, as if I were a blacksmith at Colonial Williamsburg. It's ministry as historical reenactment. They see spiritual community as a dinosaur that peaked before their parents were our age. How could it possibly be relevant to their lives? But when I talk about living a life centered on mindfulness, activism, and spiritual connection, they are intrigued.

I grew up in church, in an American Baptist church specifically, where my dad was the music director and my mom was a deacon. I left in my late teens, after surviving major depression and a handful of suicide attempts, and became an activist and a rabble-rouser. I was so angry at religion for requiring conformity of belief—why couldn't I go to church and question the doctrine? But I missed the all-ages community of congregational life. I really missed being reminded that I wasn't the center of the universe. Gaining perspective, asking hard questions. . . . Where did adults go to wonder why humans exist? To talk about what happens when we die? Without a congregation, life just seemed like small talk. Alone, I couldn't fill the hole that abandoning spirituality left behind.

Through activism, I found a spiritual community with justice at its core. Now I get to be a minister in this tradition I love that makes my life sing. I'm young, but I have experienced a lot of life: divorce, depression, abortion, friends dying, falling in and out of love. Through all of it, my spiritual communities have held me up, and so I know that church is more relevant than blacksmithing at Colonial Williamsburg. I know spiritual communities have what people are hungering for: a place to ask big questions, be accepted just as they are, and be reminded of wonder and awe.

All around me, people are busy being spiritual but not religious. I tried that for a few years myself, drawn in by the lack of required early morning activity. I read Buddhist books and practiced yoga on cold linoleum floors, joined circle dances and equinox rituals. And it was interesting, but I didn't grow. I wanted transformation, and what I got was more like a spiritual practices grab bag. But I had so many more questions. I wasn't after a prepackaged set of theology. I wanted a mystical journey, not another book to read.

Off on my mystical journey I went, on backpacking trips and in silent meditation, watching the sun rise and set. I tried to listen to that still, small voice of holiness. But I was more like Bilbo Baggins than Jesus, thinking about lunch instead of divine union, while at the same time my ego obsessed over how much weight I could lose if I skipped meditation and kept hiking. All that alone time was less about finding spiritual meaning than about me creating God in my own image.

I needed to be pushed out of my comfort zone, needed my cockiness challenged, needed people of different beliefs and backgrounds to chafe me like sand chafes a pearl. I needed a group to search alongside who would remind me that while I was a part of the universe, I wasn't the universe. I needed a spiritual community.

I spent five years pawing through the grab bag of spiritual practices before I fell in love with Unitarian Universalism. No easy answers, plenty of mystical journeying, but in partnership with other seekers. People who push me to grow while loving me just as I am. Plenty of reminders that I am not the center of the universe, plenty of time out of my comfort zone, and more pure joy than anyone expects to find on a Sunday morning. I am a part of a historic faith that is constantly changing, always adapting to fit this time and this place. I can't seem to convince anyone that worship should be in the afternoon, but otherwise I am so grateful to be spiritual and religious with my church community.

Plenty of people are mad at God because of toxic spiritual experiences from their younger days. They learned that their same-gender attraction was wrong, that Jesus cried if they masturbated, or that women need to keep their lips zipped in church. Christianity has really done a hatchet job on the psyche of many people who were dragged to church as kids. I'm really sorry if that happened to you—it sucks and it wasn't your fault and you deserved better. If anyone told you that you didn't fit into God's kingdom, they were full of shit. The spirit of love adores every inch of you, whether you are rocking the suburban working-mom life or going to amateur drag nights every night, hoping for your big break. If your minister said you weren't saved, I am sorry—they are the one who was lost. They made up a God who coincidentally shared all their bigotries. Maybe it was self-hate or maybe they just didn't have a mind big enough to take in the reality of an all-loving presence. But whatever the reason, it was their baggage. There is nothing about you that God doesn't love.

When I was eight or nine, I learned at church camp that to get an all-access pass to heaven, I needed to be saved. Being saved meant accepting Jesus, and while I thought Jesus was pretty great, I wasn't ready for an exclusive relationship with any personal Lord and savior (it's not you, Jesus, it's me). Because the version of Jesus they were selling meant no more questions. These well-meaning teenagers, charged with saving souls over summer break for minimum wage, believed that "God works in mysterious ways, so trust and be saved." And I am more the "God works in mysterious ways, so let's poke at the mystery until we get the information we're looking for" type.

The weird thing is, my religious beliefs keep saving me even though they continue to change. Jesus still saves me on a regular basis, like when I remember him saying that "the meek will inherit the earth" right before I say something snide to an authority figure. "Blessed are the peacemakers," especially those who remember not to challenge cops at protests and stay out of jail. I check in with Jesus pretty often, and so far he doesn't seem to mind that I also talk to the Buddha and Mary and my dead grandmothers. The summer camp version of Jesus was too small for me. I can't believe that our holy ones are jealous and petty. Humans have the market corned on those traits.

This book is about how my faith keeps showing up for me. It's salvific but not set. I am saved again and again without walking in lockstep with any one religious tradition. As you can read in the following chapters, I have bumbled through life making mistakes, hurting people, messing up. And yet salvation follows me, loyal and unconditionally loving. God still shows up for me, even though I am far from a faithful servant, even though I constantly have questions. I screw up, and God says, "You'll get 'em next time."

I wrote this book in order to be rich and famous— Ha, kidding! No one gets rich off writing books about spirituality. Well, except Elizabeth Gilbert, but *Eat, Pray, Love* had hot sex scenes, and this book does not. Sorry about that. But I wrote this book because spirituality is the thing I think you have been longing for, that sense of greater meaning. Wonder and awe. A sense of your place in the world that is bigger than what you do for work or what you buy or the exotic places you have traveled. You are a part of an interdependent web of all existence. You are holy and good down to your very marrow. Your resilience and kindness and patience and intellect are blowing God's mind. Did you know that? Is it time to explore it?

I don't believe in Hell, so I can't coerce you into checking out spirituality with threats of eternal damnation. But my life is roughly a trillion times better because I have faith that there is more to this life than what I can see and understand. I bet your life will be too.

1.

The Incomplete Castle

MILE-HIGH STORM CLOUDS were pushing across the sky, clear blue giving way to piles of gray and black. Long, bass-note rumbles of thunder announced the coming storm. I glanced at my brother, who was calmly piling shells into a bucket. We were building a sand castle, a huge monstrosity with towers and dungeons and, if we could figure out how, even a trap door. We spent the whole morning on the moat, making it deep enough to sink a thousand invaders, and now construction on the towers had begun. As long as this storm held off. I knew we would have to leave the beach if Mom or Dad heard that thunder, so I sped up assembly and hoped my brother would do the same.

Finishing the castle was vital, so I began to pray frantically: *Our Father who art in Heaven* . . . Whenever I felt anxious, I prayed at warp speed, saying the Lord's Prayer twenty times, then the 23rd Psalm forty times. I never stopped in the middle, and if I got interrupted, I started from the beginning, after asking God to forgive me for my distraction. My prayers became more frenzied as I saw my dad walking toward us. I needed to finish twenty rounds of both before he interrupted, or we would definitely have to go inside and abandon our castle. If I could just finish my prayers, God would send away the storm. I knew from Sunday School that God appreciated devotion—Noah built the ark, Daniel slew the lion. God rewarded his disciples' efforts. If I pleased God with my prayers, I would be allowed to finish this sand castle.

My dad sank to the sand, sitting cross-legged almost on top of our moat. He was crying. He had cried a lot lately. It terrified me, so I began another round of prayers. I started on a round of fifty *For God So Loved the World*s, silently, while Dad wept. He began to choke out apologies: he was so, so sorry. I didn't know why—we were on vacation, we were having fun. Sure, the day before, our old Chevy broke down on a busy highway. Dad had screamed so much I was surprised the car didn't start working again just to get him to be quiet. But he wasn't yelling at us, Mom said, although my brother and I were crying. He wasn't mad at us, and later we got ice cream, the blue kind with real gumballs in it. So why did he keep apologizing?

It was the family curse. I had heard the term muttered by my grandmother, "the family curse," but I didn't know what it meant. It sounded like something from a pirate story, like my ancestors had stolen a magic treasure and now we were all damned unless one of us could slay the dragon. Alas, our family curse was nothing so exciting. Our family secret is soul-sucking depression, a hopeless morass of despair that is nearly impossible to shake. The multigenerational curse of dads crying on the beach. The curse that led to suicides, aunts who never left the house, terrible tempers spinning out of anxiety attacks, dropping out, and getting fired. I wasn't the only one in the family with compulsions, who prayed frantically for a sense of control.

The family curse was real, and Dad was under its spell. Later, I would have a few turns as well, an emotional rip tide pulling me under the waves. Freeing myself took more strength than I could muster, but I was pulled from the crashing surf by the people who love me. I am broken yet beloved, imperfect but cherished. I felt them, as real as the saltwater breeze, pulling me unflaggingly through the current. I tell my story to accompany fellow travelers trying to make it back to the shore.

Back on the beach, my dad silently cried as my brother and I tried to exchange information with our eyes. Were we supposed to do something? Were there magic words to utter to dispel the curse? Then my mom was calling us inside from her perch above the beach on the motel balcony. Come in, come in. The castle abandoned, we trudged upstairs with our eyes downcast, plastic sand buckets banging against sunburned legs, wondering how long this storm would last.

2.

The Family Curse

I DON'T KNOW WHEN THE CURSE BEGAN, but my great-grandpa had it so bad he hung himself in the barn. It was the 1930s, and in New York City the stock market had crashed. The Shellabarger family farm in southern Ohio was so far away it might as well have been on another planet. Farmers rhapsodize about the soil in this part of Ohio the way folks in Napa talk about wine—it is blacker than the darkest blackberry and replete with sparkling minerals, like tiny diamonds, dumped by glaciers during the last ice age. It crumbles satisfyingly in your hand and smells like thunderstorms. In this soil grow corn and soy—crops to sell to big, faraway companies—as well as fruit for the family to enjoy: fat pink and yellow melons, bursting tomatoes, and strawberries so sweet you'd swear they were stuffed with honey.

Folks in this part of the world didn't take much notice of the goings-on in New York City. Even as the stock market

4

crashed, it didn't cause much of a stir in rural Ohio, it being the end of October and a busy time on the farm. Time to pull up the last of the year's beets, broccoli, and spinach. Bail the last fields of hay to line the barn stalls, keeping the animals warm all winter. A time for harvest festivals, pumpkin carving, and children getting new slates for school.

Over the next few years, the impact of that big-city event trickled down. Farmers were getting less for their corn and soy from the big, faraway companies. After a year of poor yields or low rates, a farmer could usually get a bank loan for seed to plant the next season, but the banks began to either shutter or not loan money to people with so little collateral. Loan officers didn't understand the value of a well-constructed barn or soil nurtured with compost for generations. Farmers seemed poor on paper, with little money in the bank.

Still, people took care of each other. Church was the center of community life, and my family were either Brethren or Mennonites, the primary difference being that Mennonites didn't allow musical instruments during worship and the Brethren did. Both churches forbade drinking, dancing, movies, playing cards, and most of all, vanity. My great-grandpa and his family were Brethren; they were willing to give up drinking and dancing, but not the old push organ wheezing out hymns like "Old Rugged Cross" on Sunday mornings.

"It's a Gift to Be Simple" was our family's favorite hymn and a communal creed. Happiness, while not strictly necessary, came from knowing you were right with God. And if you weren't right with God, you would know: crops would fail, unwed daughters would become pregnant, tumors would grow. There were no accidents. When bad things happened, it was because God was sending you a warning to change your ways. As the effects of the Great Depression reached the Ohio River Valley, folks started to wonder where they had gone wrong. Farms were repossessed. Banks put all the family's possessions out on the lawn for sale—chestnut plow horses up for auction alongside the kitchen table, the sewing machine, the German teacups from the old land, the baby's cradle. Families, now landless, stacked whatever they could fit high in the back of their pickups or hay wagons, children crying as they drove away from the fields that were meant to be their legacy, passed from generation to generation.

Fathers refused to look in the rearview mirror as they drove to the nearest big city to work in a factory. There was no word for the grief and shame of losing this family land. No memorial could encompass the feeling that you had lost what your grandparents had sacrificed to give you, that you plowed for your children's children. They didn't know that it was the scheming banks that had stolen their land, that federal farm bills had taken away their ability to make a living growing crops, had given their livelihood to big corporate conglomerates. They blamed themselves. How had they strayed from God? How could they live with their failure to hold on to the family land for the next generation?

My great-grandpa and his church friends refused to attend the bank auctions, even when good machinery was going for a pittance. They wouldn't parse over a family's belongings, wouldn't benefit from their grief. They wouldn't give a cent to the bank executives in their fancy suits, who pinched their noses at the smell of fresh manure, trying to auction off farm animals they knew nothing about, animals they wouldn't even touch with their paper-white hands. The farmers tried to save their neighbors' land, but theirs wasn't a cash economy—their wealth was in the land, in that deep black soil carrying the glittering remains of mighty glaciers. Their wealth was in healthy animals and loving children who were learning to plant and reap. Their wealth was in the church pews they built with wood they chopped down. But the banks were only interested in cash. And no one had that.

And so the bank came for my family's farm. No one knew how bad things had gotten except John, the patriarch. He had always been an anxious man, "bad nerves," they would say, but quiet, and no one worked harder. He was an exceptionally loving father—the year before, he built a cart for my grandma, his only child, Wilma. A cart with four wheels and a harness for their big golden retriever so the dog could pull her around the farm. Wilma was four and she sat proudly on her cart, thinking she looked just like her dad on his wagon, the strongest, smartest man in the world.

All around John, life was falling apart. The farm that he inherited, that he was trusted with by his father, would soon belong to strangers. Soon, the kitchen table he built, from wood that he milled, would be up for auction, alongside Wilma's toys and the chickens she lovingly fed. Soon he would work for some stranger on a factory floor, away from the pure sunlight and the precious soil that smelled like thunderstorms. How could he drive away from that farm, leaving it all behind? How could he look his wife and daughter in the eye and tell them that he had failed? The God he loved and worshipped each Sunday, the God the Brethren talk about like a friend who just stepped out of the room—how had he managed to make that God so very angry? What could he have done to cause this utter ruin?

A teenage cousin found John dangling in the barn rafters. Golden motes of dust danced in the sunlight, the barn full of the sweet scent of fresh hay. He ran to get his father, who sent for the nearest neighbor to help cut John down. For reasons lost to history, the teenage cousin was sent to get my grandmother from school. Traumatized, he stuck his head in the classroom door and said, "Come on, Wilma, we have to go. Your dad is dead. Hurry."

My great-grandpa doesn't come up in conversation much, but we all know the story: that he ended his life after learning that the farm would be repossessed. That his memorial was in the wooden church that he helped to build, his wife and daughter weeping on wooden pews made from the trees on their land. Lifelong friends unable to look them in the eye, such was the shame at a family suicide. The greatest of sins. Then the farm and the kitchen table and Wilma's little wagon and her chickens were all auctioned off by strangers in suits, turning up their noses at the manure, unable to smell the thunderstorm scent of the soil.

I grew up feeling hot anger toward my great-grandfather because the story is that he abandoned his family when life was at its worst. He left his wife and tiny daughter to fend for themselves. He brought the ultimate shame to the family: he ended his own life, he extinguished God's gift, his own creation. But now I forgive him. He was under the same family curse that I am, except he also had to face the Great Depression and this absurd idea that when bad things happened, it was because God was angry at you. I wish he knew that it was the crooked banks and not God that took his farm. I wish he lived at a time when he could get some good antianxiety medication and join a support group where men cry in front of each other and then gruffly slap each other's backs while they hug. I wish he could have kept working that magic soil, under that wide blue sky. I wish his version of God had been gentler, a God who wept with him, so he knew he wasn't alone. A God who would tell him that of course he was worthy, even without the farm. That his wife and daughter would always love him regardless. I don't know where God was on that sunny autumn day when John ended his life, but my feelings about it aren't anger anymore. Just grief.

I grieve for all that John missed: his wife starting over in a new city, finding a resilience she didn't know she contained. Wilma playing tag on urban streets with new friends, on hayrides with her high-school beaus, graduating in a smart navy suit and matching hat. Marrying a kind Brethren carpenter, building a house by his side, and raising four honest, cheerful children.

Wilma found forgiveness for her father when her own children were possessed by the family curse of depression. The understanding that mental illness is not a personal failure, not a lack of faith in the wisdom of God, but a physical ailment that tears at the victim's soul until they believe that their family would be better off without them. That it feels inescapable, that obliteration—death—feels inevitable. When it was her own son, Wilma understood. That what she had most feared—that her father didn't love her enough to fight the depression, that if she had been better he would have fought harder to live—was a dangerous mythology. That his death was the result of a long, misunderstood illness. Not a lack of love.

Depression has cursed countless generations of my family, but the mythology surrounding it will haunt us no longer. Now we separate the disease from shame. Now we talk about symptoms and medications and recovery. We feel

God standing beside us in our struggle: not in opposition, not testing us, but in loving solidarity. I wish John had lived to see it. But I feel him calling me toward resilience, toward faith, whispering in my ear: we ancestors are holding you. Never give up.

3.

Emma and Wilma

My grandmother, who was five when her dad ended his life, moved with her mother, Emma, to Dayton, the nearest city, and into the attic of her aunt Helen's house. It was just one room, with a roof that sloped low on two sides, with three flights down to the outhouse. They hung sheets across the room from a clothesline to designate rooms—an eating space, a sleeping space. My grandmother thought it was a terrific adventure, like living in a treehouse.

My great-grandmother, who had never been to a city before, talked her way into a job at a huge, stylish department store downtown. She sewed in the alterations department, and she took the trolley to work, which my grandmother found impossibly glamorous. She made half as much as the men she worked alongside, but complaining got a person fired, so she kept her complaints for home. She made just enough to get by. A kind woman in the dress department slipped Emma returned dresses that had been altered and therefore couldn't be sold, which she then resized to fit either herself or Wilma. Wilma said she was the best dressed little girl in school and that no one ever guessed they were terribly poor thanks to her trendy refitted dresses.

They didn't talk about John, ever. If they wept, they did so privately. Suicide was a sin. When Emma told people she was widowed, they were polite enough not to ask any more about it. It's hard to imagine how my grandmother and her mother dealt with this pain—John was a gentle and loving father, and they were a respected family in their small farming community. Then one day he was gone, dead by his own hand. And then the bank came for the farm, and all their familiar things were sold to strangers, and they landed in a busy loud city. Friends were far away, their church was far away, and John was never coming back. How does a five-year-old cope with all of that? How did she know not to mention her dad, not to ask questions? I wonder if church brought her any relief. As soon as they moved to Dayton, Emma and Wilma started attending Helen's Church of the Brethren congregation, a more liberal outpost of the denomination than the one they attended in the country.

My grandmother's Aunt Helen was married to an "old cuss who didn't even go to church," Grandma said, not going to church being a sin just short of murder in her mind. He wanted to rent the attic to paying tenants and was miffed that his wife's sister was living there for free. He constantly threatened to kick them out, but Helen was kind and adored my grandmother. Helen would make a huge dinner, much too big for just her and her husband, and then say, "Oh well, I guess I'll take the leftovers upstairs." When her husband started yelling that he wasn't working to feed her widowed sister, Helen started making dinner just for herself, Emma, and Wilma. She took it up to them and told him she hadn't had time to make his dinner. After enough ham sandwiches and cold canned beans for supper, he begged forgiveness.

After a dozen or so years, Emma had scraped together enough money to buy a home. She and Wilma shared a room while renting out the other bedrooms to boarders. My great-grandmother was one of the few people in Dayton who would rent to Japanese Americans during World War II, saying that since she had no control over what the men in Washington, D.C., did, she imagined that Japanese Americans certainly didn't have any control over what Japanese leaders were up to. Why demonize thousands of people based on the decisions of a few men? She befriended many Japanese American families, and my grandma knew a more diverse range of people than her classmates. This didn't make them popular in their neighborhood. Anti-Japanese sentiment was high, especially as more and more boys died in the war. But the exhaustion of working for her own living and the independence of heading her own family had formed Emma into a woman who didn't care what other people thought.

Soon Emma had enough money to buy a real boarding house full of young men that she bossed about, making them fix things around the house in addition to paying rent. She had a reputation for being formidable but fair. She eventually had enough money to retire, a happy ending to what could have been a lifetime of poverty. She never remarried, and I don't know if she ever forgave her husband. I don't know if she agreed with the church that suicide earns a person a place in Hell, even if they were very kind, even if they built the very pews in the sanctuary and a little dog cart for their daughter. I hope she forgave him. I hope she knew that God was bigger and better than a rigid, legalistic judge doling out damnation. That God knows that an awful symptom of depression is believing that the world would be better if you didn't exist, that your family would be better off without you. That John was just awfully sick with depression, and it wasn't that he didn't love her and Wilma.

Everything I know about John I learned from Wilma, who talked about him in a disappointed way—her dad, the strongest, kindest man in the world, who left her. Abandoned her to poverty. She said very little about him, her hands twisting into fists. Then she would sigh and say that she sure had a lot of questions for God when she got to heaven. She would wring her small hands and say that she sure wanted to know why things worked the way they did. And then, still a farmer at heart, she would dust her hands off on her trousers and get back to work in the garden, pulling weeds and picking cucumbers.

I don't know why we are born or what happens when we die, I don't know why depression exists or why unfettered greed was allowed to take away the livelihoods of millions during the Great Depression. I do know that we have a choice: believe in a God who is ultimately powerful, or ultimately loving. Anyone who has loved a person with depression knows that we can't have both—a God who loved us and controlled everything wouldn't let depression exist. Or childhood cancers, or earthquakes, or hangnails. Definitely not mosquitoes. God is either our dear partner in our struggles or the reason for those struggles.

I reject the God who gives us what we deserve, who keeps a tally of right-doings and wrongdoings and doles out punishments for every single sin. The God John believed in only sent a person what they earned through good works or errant living. I have so much in my life I didn't earn: kind parents, good physical health, free public school education. Beethoven, Joni Mitchell, and Beyoncé. Libraries, national parks, and street festivals. Bursting red tomatoes, buttery sweet corn, and succulent pink watermelons. Thank goodness I haven't gotten what I deserve. Many are less fortunate. I don't believe God loves them any less than he loves me.

This is the struggle that most of us have with God. How can the God who created tiny baby toes and tangerine-orange sunsets have also made childhood cancer? If God is an endless fount of compassion, why is there famine? Child soldiers, AIDS, sexual assault, addiction? Why would the God who loves us make life so damn hard?

For me, God—whom I prefer to call Goddess, or Luna, or Love, just to disrupt the male-God dominance we have faced for eight thousand years—isn't a creature or a supernatural person. God isn't Mr. Rogers or Santa Claus in the sky (but if God did have to be a man, Mr. Rogers would be a great choice). God is a force, a push to do what is loving. God is the voice that urges us to forgive. God is a piece of every living creature, the best piece, the part that connects us. The part that makes us brave enough to embrace each other. God is always cheering on anyone struggling, anyone who feels hopeless. God is my ancestors whispering, "Hang in there. You are stronger than you know. It only gets better up ahead," in my ear when I think the depression will never end.

Perhaps this seems too good to be true. On my more cynical days, I wonder if it is a little too convenient. It feels too easy to let God off the hook for famine, for addiction, for AIDS. Too easy to assume God is with the oppressed as they are shoved down again and again. If God loves them so damn much, why do they continue to suffer? If God loves all of us so damn much, why do any of us suffer?

My friend, the radical Reform rabbi I go to for spiritual wisdom, says that the human brain only recognizes contrast. Without hot, we don't understand cold. Without hunger, we don't understand feeling fed. So God allows us to suffer—not creating suffering, we do that perfectly well on our own—so we can feel the euphoria of not suffering. Maybe so. I'm not sure about that one. As I have mentioned before, "I'm not sure" is an acceptable statement in my faith tradition. We are proudly agnostic, letting our beliefs evolve as we experience the world.

I am sure that what we think about God impacts how we treat each other. If we believe that every person gets what they deserve, that God is tallying every sin and sending an equal punishment, then we are unlikely to sympathize with someone who is suffering. If we think that John lost his farm because he did enough wrong to earn that punishment, we are unlikely to help him. We are unlikely to be compassionate. We are more likely to keep score of each other's sins and dole out the punishments we think will even the scales. As if we are God ourselves. As if our own lives are without sin.

If we believe that God is sitting beside us in our suffering, that God is urging us to be loving—whispering that we should turn toward justice, pressuring us to be compassionate—we are more likely to put an arm around John's shoulders. Help him move away from shame and through his grief. On a bigger scale, we are more apt to fight the types of financial injustices that led to the Great Depression and to advocate for just banking practices. Because the way we think about God—whether it is the

Santa Claus God of childhood, the ticked-off God of Noah's flood, or the energy of compassion that moves among us— affects how we treat each other. Our feelings about God color our every encounter, from the voting booth to how we treat the checkout clerk at the gas station. What we think about God matters.

It is unlikely that we will have any definite answers about the nature of God in this lifetime. As my Grandma Wilma always said, I sure have a lot of questions for God. Maybe we won't even get the answers we want after we die. But I choose to believe in the God who makes me kinder. Because no one knows for sure who or what God is, so why choose a bully keeping accounts of every sin? I choose the God of compassion who sits beside me when I weep and pushes me to comfort the troubled.

4.

It's All Jimmy Carter's Fault

MY GRANDMOTHER WILMA married a man just like her dad—which drove her mom Emma nuts, but what can you do? Wilma was a rebellious teenager, going to movies, which Brethren were not supposed to do. At least Leonard was a nice boy from church. He was a hard worker. But like John, he had the curse, the sadness that obliterates reality. The anxiety that uncorks as rage. Leonard was a gentle soul until the minute he lost his temper. Then fury took over his mind and he screamed louder than thunder. He was a man possessed and could not be calmed until his energy ran out and he collapsed.

In my family, at least, this is how anxiety works: men don't know how to cope with panic attacks, so they rage, taking out their anger on whoever is nearby. Women turn the fear inward and become depressed. We weep to the point of incapacitation. There are certainly gender norms at play here—women don't rage because women aren't supposed to get angry. Society punishes women who express anger. But women are allowed to feel sad, so that is how the anxiety expresses itself. Societal norms say men aren't supposed to cry, but they are allowed to take out their feelings on other people. So out comes their rage. One gendered response isn't better than another—and, of course, not everyone's anxiety manifests this way. Either way, the anxiety is being released in an unhealthy way. Either way there is suffering. I cry when I'm anxious, but I also pray compulsively—not particularly heartfelt prayer, but speed-recitation of memorized prayers like "The Lord Is My Shepherd." As far as I know, I'm the only one with a compulsive praying coping strategy, but it isn't much of a surprise in a super-religious family like mine.

Wilma and Leonard had four children, the third of whom is my dad, Ray. Ray inherited the family curse, as did all four kids, to differing extents. Ray hid his anxiety behind anger, like his dad, hollering like thunder in the same key as Leonard. His sisters hid from his rages, his mom rolled her eyes at having two yellers in the house. I doubt anyone ever suggested that there was a better way to cope with mental illness, since "mental illness" wasn't a term people used and no one was admitting to how awful they felt, lest they end up in a looney bin. No one was admitting to the waves of terror that come with a panic attack—the fear over nothing at all, the strangling sensation, the heart-exploding feeling, the claustrophobia. Sadly, a house full of people were all having panic attacks and pretending that they were fine, lest people think they were crazy.

They all thought they were the only ones with the curse that killed Grandpa John. Grandpa John, the man who abandoned his family, lost them the farm, and committed the gravest sin. Everyone feared, but no one admitted, that they were like him. They were scared that they, too, might submit to the madness and end up hanging from the rafters. But no one spoke of it.

When my dad was in his early twenties and student teaching, the anxiety became too much to bear. His principal said he couldn't yell at students so often, and he was crying a lot at home. He felt sick with hot shame—what if he couldn't teach? What if he couldn't work at all? He felt broken. His friends were off fighting in Vietnam, and he couldn't even handle student teaching? He felt guilty for feeling anything other than grateful not to be at war in a faraway jungle. And yet he wept whenever he was alone and shook with fear.

He went to the family doctor, who first assumed he was a shell-shocked vet. Returning soldiers had similar struggles, but no one was talking about anxiety disorders outside of the military. Decades before, Freud wrote about childhood trauma leading to adult neurosis, but my dad didn't consider his childhood traumatic. Sure, his dad was calm one moment and furious the next. Sure, his big sister was so shaken by Leonard screaming at her while teaching her to drive that even now, in her seventies, she refuses to drive. But what was traumatic about that?

The doctor didn't have any treatments for my dad, who had hoped to hear that he just needed a shot of something or another and then he could be normal. He prescribed heavy-duty sedatives and told Dad to work more so he had less time to think about his problems. This idea, that anxiety and depression can be cured by just thinking less and staying busy, comes up all the time, even now, when people recommend that a depressed person just volunteer at the hospital so they can see how bad other people have it, as if depressed people are just spoiled brats who are bored into sadness. It's impossible to miss the judgment in the doctor's words—if you had to work hard, if you were at war like all the other men your age, you certainly wouldn't have time to have these silly issues. Chin up, soldier!

So began Ray's on-and-off use of sedatives. He couldn't take them all the time—on them, he could barely stay awake, hardly control a classroom, just manage to eke out a full sentence or two. He bloated up in weight and fell asleep at Sunday dinner. Without them, he had panic attacks. A reduced dosage didn't do anything at all. So he only took them when the anxiety was truly unbearable or when he couldn't stop crying after a few hours.

I have no idea how my dad managed to convince my mom to marry him while in this either-dopey-or-panicking state, but he did. They were both working second jobs at Christmastime, holiday employees at the huge, glamorous department store that anchored downtown Dayton in the 1970s. At the end of the night, they had to count the cash in their registers. My dad counted out loud, which drove my mom nuts because then she would lose her count. So she snapped at him a few times, and somehow that made him want to go out with her, and a year later they were married.

A year after that, I was born, thanks to Jimmy Carter, the peanut-farmer-turned-president. My parents didn't plan to have children. The world in the late 1970s was too bleak. There were race riots in our town. Nuclear winter felt imminent; it would wipe out humanity before a child of theirs would have a chance to grow up. It would be cruel to bring a child into the violence and chaos. Plus, my dad was depressed or anxious a lot of the time, and Mom liked her job and didn't want to be a stay-at-home-mom. Stay-at-home-dads weren't a thing in Dayton yet.

And then came a peanut farmer who taught Sunday school, despised warfare, and stared at his wife with so much love you'd think they were newlyweds. My parents, Jesus- and Joan Baez–loving do-gooders, thought that if Jimmy Carter could be elected president, maybe this world wasn't damned after all. Maybe there was hope for another generation.

I was born, and less than two years later, my brother followed. We were only a few years old when Carter was unseated by Reagan, whom my dad referred to, mostly joking, as the anti-Christ. By then it was too late to go back to not having kids, and fortunately my parents thought having children was pretty fun.

Could two children have been treasured any more? Every day, my dad came home for lunch and sang, "K-k-k Katie, beautiful Katie, I'll be waiting for you at the kitchen door," while dancing me around the room. I thought he made that song up for me until late elementary school, when I heard it on a record at school. Talk about disappointment! But my parents delighted in spending time with us, reading us children's Bible stories, walking to the park nearby to swing, and making up silly, complicated stories on long car rides.

We had an idyllic, pre-Internet, pre–video games childhood, watching *Sesame Street* on one of the three channels our TV received while eating sugary breakfast cereal, then running outside to tear up and down the street with a pack of other neighborhood kids until Mom hollered at us to come in for lunch meat sandwiches. Mom didn't go back to work until I started kindergarten, and in my few recollections of that time, she is tall, tan, and smiling, always soft-voiced, pulling me in for millions of hugs with her baby-oiled arms. My mom had a large mole on her face, right between her eyebrows, and even now, when I see a woman with a mole, I think she is so beautiful. Do all children think their mother is the prettiest? I remember thinking other mothers didn't smell as good as mine, with her sweet, sweaty scent. First thing in the morning, her breath was like sourdough bread and I loved it. When my parents went out on a date, she wore Chanel Number Five and a red dress, and I thought she looked like a movie star. I secretly worried that she would be discovered by a big Hollywood agent and fame would sweep her away from us.

Life with my dad was more complicated. There was no middle ground, no regular time. Life was either perfect or a disaster, and Dad's depression and anger kept us teetering. When he was happy, he coached our soccer teams, helped build our science fair projects, and led sing-alongs at Girl Scout camp. He built bonfires in the backyard so we could roast marshmallows. He had endless time and patience for all the duties of being a dad and seemed to really enjoy it. All of my school friends thought he was perfect.

Until he was angry. His moods were unpredictable, and we didn't know what to expect when he came home—would he tease us, tickle us, read us bedtime stories using funny voices? Would he yell and slam things around? Would Mom scuttle about trying to appease him, or would she become angry too and argue? It was a terrible adventure that made my stomach heave and heart flutter. Who would Dad be when he got home? Mr. Rogers or Freddie Kruger?

My dad is a musician and often had rehearsals or concerts in the evenings. My mom would get angry and say he only cared about performing, not about us. He would stomp out of the house, slamming the doors. He got mad for other reasons too, reasons I didn't understand. He was a paid soloist at our church and he would often come home from church angry. I tried to control his temper by praying obsessively, saying the Lord's Prayer forty times. I made millions of deals with God: if Dad would stay happy, I wouldn't think any mean thoughts about my brother. I would let him play with my toys. I would be patient. It didn't work, either me being patient or Dad staying happy. Home was an anxious and unhappy place when he was upset. I spent a lot of time thinking about when Dad came home, torn between excitement at possibly seeing my smiling, goofy dad and fear that he would slam the door and swear.

My dad fell into depressions that sometimes lasted for months. He didn't dance me around or throw the softball with us; he didn't want to wrestle or play games. He rarely even made eye contact. He yelled more. I remember laughing when I heard the phrase "don't cry over spilled milk," because Tom or me spilling milk at dinner was a major problem when my dad was sad. He would yell and fume, then apologize, and sometimes cry right there in front of us. It was awful. Worst of all, sometimes I could hear him crying in the basement or in my parents' room late at night. The sobs sounded like they were being squeezed out of him, painfully, involuntarily. Like he was in agony.

I love my parents and feel lucky to be their kid. They were good parents, whatever that means, but depression and anxiety are hard to explain to a child. I don't think there was a specific way my parents "should" have explained the crying and the rages to me, but some information would have been helpful. So that I didn't try to fix it myself. So my brother and I didn't wonder if it was our fault.

In an ideal world, dads wouldn't have rage problems and chronic depression. There was no Little Golden Book to explain my dad's weeping. There were times in my childhood when my dad was suicidal, and my mom reminded him, "You can't commit suicide and mess up the kids' lives," like a mantra. I feel lucky that he didn't end his life, that he had the tenacity to stay with us even when there was no relief from the despair. For decades he suffered without therapy, medication, or even knowing that his mental illness was an illness and not his fault. Decades of guilt and shame. Decades of being afraid he wouldn't ever feel better, that he might not be able to parent, to support the family financially. How did he keep going? Where does that amazing resilience come from?

I feel lucky that my dad worked for the city government and had health benefits that included the emerging field of behavioral health. When I was a teenager in the early 1990s, behavioral health wasn't a field anyone was talking about in southern Ohio. Mental problems were to be solved with prayer and willpower, or more likely not solved at all. But my dad overcame the stigma and started seeing a psychologist and a mental health counselor. His rages became farther and farther apart, and he began to cope with his anxiety in healthier ways. Dad became the kind of sensitive guy who talks about his feelings, who can apologize and repair a relationship instead of just stomping off.

Best of all, he became the kind of guy who talks publicly and without shame about having mental illness. It was wildly unusual that he was going to therapy at all, much less talking about it. But Dad told everyone—people at work, people at church, our neighbors, my friends' parents. He became the number one fan of mental health services.

My childhood was weird, but doesn't everyone feel that way? There was tremendous joy, like when my dad sang and danced me around the room. There was tremendous anxiety, wondering if Dad would be mad when he came home. I feel grateful to my parents for loving Tom and me so abundantly. There was not one second of my childhood when I doubted that they were crazy about me. And I'm grateful that my dad was so open about his mental illness, because stigmas are hard, but secrets are awful. Too many generations suffered the family curse in silence. My dad was the first to speak up, and he spoke loudly.

5.

Choose Jesus . . . or Else

When I was a little girl, I loved summer camp. Canoeing on a lake covered with slimy moss, flipping the boat and coming up with algae in my hair. Weaving God's Eyes from two sticks and red, orange, and yellow yarn, the same colors as the sunset. Tucked into my sleeping bag in my cabin, on the top bunk, listening to the crickets. Camp felt like the best place in the whole world. And sure, sometimes it was a little scary. It was pitch black at night. There were owls in the trees and coyotes wailing nearby. But every evening, the campfire made a golden orb in the mysterious darkness, a place safe from wild animals and ghosts. When I was inside that circle, I was cozily sandwiched by friends sitting on either side of me on a scratchy log. I was inside of the orb, and the fire was warm and the smell of bug spray was heavy and we sang songs about Jesus and God and heaven, and all was right with the world.

Did I mention this was church camp? Baptist church camp? I was raised in a liberal American Baptist church, but this camp was a free-for-all of Baptists from all over the state: Southern Baptists, evangelical Baptists. And that didn't really matter to me—kids are kids, and God didn't come up much during crafts and capture the flag. But every night at campfire, after we sang our silly songs with huge hand gestures— Jesus is a rock and he rolls my blues away, bop shu bop bop shu bop—we would have a little sermon. Most nights, this sermon covered pretty obvious stuff: be nice to each other; Jesus said so. Don't covet other people's stuff; the Ten Commandments said so. But one evening, things became more serious. Words I didn't hear much in my church started popping up during the sermon: salvation, damnation, Hell, being saved. And I became more aware of the darkness outside the cozy camp circle—the unending blackness, pierced only by the licking golden flames of the fire.

It was time to declare our commitment to God, the camp minister said, to Jesus. Tonight was the night. It was time to be saved. And one by one, as the teenage camp counselors sang a weepy song to us, my camp friends came forward to accept Jesus as their personal lord and savior and take communion. Soon the ten-year-old girls sitting on either side of me were up front, and I was the only one sitting on my log. And then the only kid still sitting on any log.

And then they were all staring, waiting—why wasn't I coming forward? I can't say exactly why I didn't move. In my liberal congregation, kids started talking about getting baptized around thirteen; it was an older kid thing. It was a serious rite, but it was optional and there was no pressure. This way was pretty alien to me—it seemed exploitive, although I didn't know that word at the time. It felt like I was being peer pressured into a personal relationship with Jesus. I liked Jesus quite a bit, and I didn't have any objection to getting saved eventually. But this was weird. Coercive, with the mushy singing and the threat of Hell so easy to imagine in the dark woods. Maybe the devil was real; maybe he was right out there, two feet past our lit circle.

So I didn't stand up, even when the camp minister talked more about Hell and salvation, even when he asked me directly, "Aren't you worried that you'll die in your sleep and end up in Hell? Just because you didn't accept Jesus tonight? Because none of us knows when we will die, but we do know that without Jesus, we are going to burn for eternity." Well, sure, I was worried, and thanks a lot for bringing up both death and Hell when I am in the woods, far from home, in the middle of the night. But I stayed in my seat. It just didn't feel right.

And finally, after a few more verses of the mushy Jesus song, after a few more "last chances," the campfire was over, and we clustered and headed into the dark, back to our cabin. Then my cabin's camp counselor pulled me aside, one on one. "Don't you think it hurts Jesus, hurts his feelings, when you turn away like that? Jesus just wants you in his kingdom." I just shook my head and headed to my bunk.

It was a long night, hours of being afraid to fall asleep because I might die and go to Hell. But by morning the fear had turned to confusion—this wasn't the Jesus I knew. This wasn't the God I knew. Could the adults have it wrong on this one? I loved a man called Jesus who fed strangers with miraculously multiplying fish and bread. Jesus didn't ask for a firm faith commitment from all who came to eat, he just fed them. Who was this Jesus who consigned little girls to Hell because they didn't participate in the communion feast of a square of white bread and paper cup of sweet grape juice? Because they didn't feel ready at that very minute and then dropped dead? No, I couldn't see Jesus damning me by technicality.

It worried me, though, this idea that Jesus might be sore because I didn't come forward at the campfire. I liked Jesus. I pictured him playing the acoustic guitar and looking forlorn, like a hippie whose girlfriend just dumped him. Was I breaking Jesus' heart?

The next day my parents came to pick me up and I told them the whole story. They exchanged a lot of raised-eyebrow looks in the front seat, and a few "Did you know it was *that* kind of church camp?" remarks. They told me Jesus didn't get mad at children ("But he sure should be pissed at that camp minister," my dad muttered under his breath). Jesus and God loved every person in the whole world, unconditionally. I countered, "But what about heaven?" Mom replied, "Everyone is going to heaven. God loves people too much to send anyone to Hell. Hell isn't real."

I wasn't so sure about that. At church, we didn't talk about Hell. Lots about Jesus healing the sick and feeding the poor. I knew the Beatitudes ("Blessed are the weak . . .") backward and forward. But I hadn't heard about damnation. Nevertheless, at camp we talked about Hell constantly—who was going, who wasn't. I learned that whole countries were going to Hell because people there believed in different gods, the wrong gods. Kids born in those countries didn't even have a shot at heaven, my camp counselor said. Think how lucky we are, she said, to be raised in the right religion.

Reporting this to my parents caused them to sigh a lot and say maybe next year Girl Scout camp would be a better choice. Mom said, "Everyone thinks their religion is the right one, the only real one. But sweetie, no one knows. We just have to try to be good people and trust that God loves us all." That was a lot of information to consider: no one knows what is real about God?! It ran counter to everything I'd heard at camp all week. At camp we were the very few and very blessed, selected for a very exclusive trip to heaven. But the way my mom was talking, the whole world would be up there.

I'm lucky I had parents who talked about religion. Kids hear so much, way more than parents realize, about God,

Hell, Jesus, the whole theological rigmarole. From evangel-icals at camp, from children at school, from well-meaning adults who want to save their souls by scaring them into taking Jesus into their hearts. Christianity by coercion. Lots of kids were like me, terrified of Hell, confused about Christ, and anxious about screwing up the afterlife before we'd even reached adulthood. Worrying about my dad coming home angry and yelling about spilled milk was nothing com-pared to worrying about God being angry and sending me to eternal torment. Thank goodness my parents talked openly about religion. I knew faith was a topic I could bring up.

Oddly, the solution to all this anxiety caused by mis-information about God is more church, more synagogue, more time at the mosque, more talking to kids about reli-gion. Kids are curious about much more than they will ask about—what happens after death, why bad things happen to good people, where we come from, why we are born. What they hear from kids and adults outside of their family can terrify them. Going to a liberal congregation where questions are welcomed and fear isn't wielded to force belief means kids learn to think critically about religion. They start to figure out what they believe in and what they do not.

If parents don't bring up faith, kids hear horror stories about Hell and damnation. Homophobic and transphobic ideas about "Adam and Eve, not Adam and Steve." Racist ideas about the wholesale damnation of people in other countries who refuse to submit to the invasion of Christian missionaries. A vacuum will be filled. Just like the birds and the bees talk, faith can be an awkward topic, but children wonder about religion and are searching for answers.

I know some grown-ups think they are doing kids a favor by not putting them through the stultifying sermons they endured as children or the hate-filled religious rhetoric that emotionally scarred them. I am not suggesting sending your kid off to the fundamentalists every week. But they need to hear about religion from adults they can trust. At a minimum, that means checking in with them every month to see what they've heard about God. Maybe it means taking them to a liberal congregation where they can hear about a loving God, learn about the holy scriptures in their historical context, and practice thinking critically about the ways people use the idea of God to hurt each other. Because kids are hearing and thinking about faith. It just might be scaring the hell out of them.

After talking to my parents (and following up with my Sunday school teachers, just to verify), I went back to being comfortably sure that God, Jesus, and I were on positive terms. I wasn't sure about all the details: being saved, getting baptized, sin and salvation. But in my mind, I was still in the golden orb of the campfire, in the warmth of God's love, despite the fundamentalist grown-ups' attempts to tell me otherwise.

6.

Sadness the Chimp and the Evil Katieo

NO ONE WANTS TO BE the villain in their own story. I bet Judas didn't wake up thinking, "Hey, I think I'll turn Jesus in to the bad guys today and then be hated for the next two millennia. I hope people curse my name long after I'm dead!" But I am trying to tell my story as best I can, and so I can't leave out that I was Lex Luthor to my brother's Superman.

I was jealous of my brother the second I met him at the hospital when I was eighteen months old. I don't care if science says I can't possibly remember anything that happened when I was that young—I remember meeting that little bundle of joy and thinking the gravy train was over. No more would I be the super-special, overly adored only child. Soon, my made-up songs—my parents loved my nonsense songs!—were too loud, the baby was sleeping. Soon my grandparents, who as far as I knew were full-time Katie fans, were cooing over the baby. Stupid baby.

It didn't help that Tom has these bright blue eyes that twinkle annoyingly, like the lead in a Hallmark romantic comedy. When he was little, our daycare teachers called him Tommy Blue Eyes and Tommy Cookie ("because he's so sweet!"). They called me Katie. Just Katie. Occasionally Katie-why-don't-you-let-someone-else-talk-for-a-while or Katie-we-don't-sing-and-dance-during-naptime. But no cutesy terms of endearment about my slightly crossed brown eyes covered with pink plastic glasses. I had full-scale jealous big sister syndrome. When he was sleeping, I would sneak up to his crib and pinch his cheeks until he cried. Take that, Tommy Blue Eyes. When he was learning to walk, I knocked him over. By the time he started school, he was plaintively asking, "Why do you hate me?"

And he wasn't just cuter than me, he was smarter too. In kindergarten, Tom solved my Rubik's cube and then gave me this "What, are these supposed to be hard?" look. We learned to read at the same time (he was three!), and he could ride his bike without training wheels months before I could. But I was outgoing and he was shy. I was busy singing the entire Annie soundtrack to anyone who would listen, complete with original hand motions and costume changes. Surely that equaled his ability to solve the problems in my math book. Tommy and I were different, but he wasn't better than me. Until he officially became Gifted.

When I was in third grade, we moved to the suburbs and started at a new school. Tom was in first grade and was quickly awarded entry to the gifted and talented program. I didn't even know there was a gifted and talented program, but apparently it involved field trips, so I wanted in. I asked my parents to sign me up. My poor parents—how do you explain to one of your kids that they have already been deemed not good enough? That they have already been weeded out of the "special" group? I don't know what they said—it was probably very gentle and kind—but I recall how I felt.

Shame. Hot, violent, shame rose up through my torso. I thought I was going to vomit it up, this awful, physical sensation lurching around my body. I ran to the bathroom and knelt over the toilet to expel the comet of hate pummeling my every limb. But it wouldn't come out. The feelings were stuck inside of me. I hated myself. I was stupid. Shame: a brand-new feeling. It felt horrible. How could I get it out?

I scored my arms and legs with my fingernails, trying to give the hate a way to escape through my skin, but it brought no relief. I started to scream and cry and lunged onto my brother, knocking him to the floor, hitting him. Then I saw how scared he looked, how confused. He hadn't taunted me or bragged; he didn't ask to be in the gifted program. I loved him so much and I was hurting him for being smart. If I was a good sister, I would be happy for him. I was bad. Stupid and mean. I ran to my room and locked the door, crying and scratching my skin until bright red stripes covered me. The shame swirled, peaking and abating in rapid cycles. Exhausted and out of tears to cry, I finally fell asleep.

The next day at school I had a bright yellow note taped to my desk: an appointment with the guidance counselor. My parents had called in the professionals for backup. Soon I was sitting sulkily across from kindly Mr. Dotsam in his stuffed animal–filled office. He was gently trying to get me to stop hating my brother and myself. We talked about how different people are good at different things and how school doesn't test everything. That I was good at things outside of school, like ballet dancing and Girl Scouts, that my brother didn't participate in at all. We talked about how every person needs to know, deep down, that they are good enough; that they are worthy, even when they don't get good grades or have twinkly blue eyes. He told me that after I got out of school, I would find that grades didn't matter much at all.

It helped a lot. I didn't really get the self-worth-no-matter-what piece, but I was only eight. Monks spend lifetimes trying to torch their needy egos; I had time to work on it. I understood that I was good at things Tommy wasn't good at, and that being bad at school didn't mean I would be bad at being an adult. An official school-approved adult said I was good enough. But I still felt ashamed, and I continued to try to expel my shame by hurting Tom.

I struggled in school, barely making Cs. Not a single subject came easily to me. I spent hours on incomprehensible worksheets that my brother completed on our fifteen-minute ride home on the school bus. I had math tutoring every Saturday morning while my brother stayed home and watched cartoons. Meanwhile, my math teacher asked why I couldn't just ask my brother for help (I'm guessing she didn't have siblings). I couldn't understand why school was easy for Tom—it felt like it was easy for everybody but me. Was I stupid? Would I be stupid if annoying Tommy wasn't around to make me look bad? It had to be his fault. Otherwise I was a defective person. Before he was born, I was special. I was adored! It was his fault.

When I was around ten and he around eight, we drove all the way from Ohio to the Grand Canyon. What I remember is the blast of heat I felt when I opened the car door to get in, fast food smells, and candy melted to the floor of the car. I remember secretly filling an empty paper bag with red dirt in Kentucky while my parents gassed up the car. It was such a crazy color! Like Mars! But it was also full of red ants, the kind that bite, and twenty miles down the highway we realized that they were all over us. Thank goodness for car wash vacuums and calamine lotion.

What the rest of my family remembers from our Grand Canyon road trip is that my brother drew comic strips in the car, short storylines with brutal, cartoon-style violence, a ruthless villain, and an innocent victim who never saw justice. The cartoons were titled *Sadness the Chimp and the Evil Katieo*. And, surprise, surprise, Sadness looked just like a monkey version of my brother, and the Evil Katieo had glasses and long, straight hair like me.

The plotlines followed this formula: Sadness the Chimp was doing something sweet like picking flowers or making cookies for his friends. Then the Evil Katieo would enter the scene, destroy whatever Sadness was doing, and knock him over the head. Katieo would laugh maniacally at her destruction and leave happy. Sadness would cry pitifully. The end. No justice. The Evil Katieo was never punished. Sadness never found a way to defend himself.

It doesn't take a psychiatrist to interpret Tom's feelings. When I got mad about the comics, he said they weren't about me, that the Evil Katieo was just a made-up name. Little liar. And if the comics were a cry for help directed at my parents, I don't think it worked. They found the whole thing hilarious, not concerning.

But why was I so mad at Tom? Sure, there was sibling rivalry, combined with jealousy at his being an academic superstar. He is exceptionally bright: in eighth grade he took college physics for fun. He read encyclopedias in his spare time. He got scholarships to MIT and Caltech. Now he has a degree in nuclear physics. I text him when I need to divide fractions for a recipe (he tells me that I can use

Google to figure it out, but it's easier to ask him. I should get something out of his braininess). Sharing parents with a genius would be a lot for any sibling.

But I was also a kid with an undiagnosed anxiety disorder and a sad and angry dad. At home, the unspoken but apparent rule was that Dad was the only one allowed to have problems, especially emotional problems. My husband is a mental health therapist, and he tells me this is called "identified patient syndrome." When one person in a family is struggling with something big—illness, addiction, that kind of thing—everyone else gets into a supportive role around them. A family concentrating their energy on one person works well during a crisis; if Mom breaks a leg and everyone rallies to take care of her, that is a good way for kids to learn responsibility and everyone to grow closer. Problems arise, however, when the patient has a chronic, long-term illness like my dad's depression and anxiety. Then other family members don't feel like there is enough energy left over to handle their own needs. My dad struggled and we love him, so we formed a web of care around him. It wasn't out of obligation but a show of affection and loyalty. But the web lasted for decades because his illness lasted for decades. It is stressful for a kid to be a part of an adult's unspoken care system. It also meant I didn't feel like I could ask for help because the family's energy was already committed to helping Dad.

Nobody ever said out loud that Dad was our identified patient. My parents were and are loving, caring people. But maintaining Dad's equanimity was time- and energy-intensive. So I didn't feel like there was space for me to ask for help, much less know how to ask for help with a problem I didn't know how to name. My shame and rage at my brother's acceptance to the gifted program were probably my first panic attack, and they came regularly for the rest of my childhood. But I didn't know how to name what was happening, a stomachache mixed with fear mixed with despair. I didn't know that was called a panic attack; I just knew it felt like the world was ending. But Dad was the one with problems, not me.

There was also no space for expressing how helpless I felt about my poor academics. My grades got even worse as I entered high school; my math teacher said I wasn't college material and should consider cosmetology school. I couldn't even master feathering my own hair, much less anyone else's. The future seemed bleak. I was too anxious to learn anything—math or hair feathering, it was all drowned out by the furious beat of my panicked heart. The anxiety took up all my energy, and nothing was left for learning.

The day I turned sixteen, I got a job waiting tables at a local diner and wondered if that would be my career path. But I was terrible at waitressing too. It was hard to remember that table nine needed coffee creamer when I was in the middle of an anxiety attack. During the lunch and dinner rush I would start to shake with anxiety, which didn't bode well for the big plates of spaghetti I was delivering. I ruined many a customer's shirt before I was fired.

But by then Sadness the Chimp, otherwise known as Tom, was finished being victimized. Soon after our Grand Canyon road trip, he began practicing martial arts. I learned quickly that if I lunged at him, he could grab my arm and neatly flip me over his head. It didn't hurt, but it was unnerving after all those years of being bigger and stronger than him. Fighting my brother wasn't a good idea anymore. I found myself surprisingly relieved by this end to the violence I precipitated. The guilt I felt after pummeling him, the damage to our sibling relationship—it wasn't worth it.

My jealousy began to abate as we shared friends in high school, and I began to see him as a whole person instead of just my rival, a rival who always won. He wasn't just smart; he was funny, and had hopeless crushes on my friends, and even had the occasional zit. He even helped me with my math homework without making a big deal about it, without teasing me even a little. I loved my brother from the moment I met him, but I didn't really know him until we were teenagers.

Now Tom and I are buddies, even though he is still annoyingly handsome and smart. It's irritating, but I love him anyway. And he is one of those secretly nice people. For example, if I volunteer at a homeless shelter, I tell everyone. I humble brag so hard. "Did I mention that I got a speeding ticket on my way to volunteer at the homeless shelter?" Everything I say for months will somehow involve my mentioning my volunteering. "Did you try the new

Korean restaurant on First Ave.? They have really spicy kimchi and it's right by the homeless shelter where I volunteered that one time three years ago." But Tom never mentions when he does something for someone else. I only found out he was donating blood because he fainted after his ten billionth withdraw and the nurse called my mom, who was still listed as his emergency contact.

If I could go back and change one thing in my life, it would be bullying Tommy Blue Eyes. I was terrible to my only sibling, my closest relative. I was Cruella de Vil to all the cute puppies; I was Stalin in pink footie pajamas. I don't want that meanness to be a part of my history, of who I am. I don't want the fear and confusion of having a spiteful big sister to be a part of my brother's history, a part of who he is now. He forgives me, but it still happened. Neither of us can forget it. Can I forgive myself?

Luckily, I have a lot of spiritual help around forgiveness. Growing up in the American Baptist tradition, we said the Lord's Prayer every week. It includes this religious gem: Forgive us our debts, as we forgive those who debt against us. (I know some congregations say, "Forgive us our trespasses, as we forgive those who trespass against us." Baptists aren't so fancy-pants with their language.) For as long as I can remember, standing in the pew between my mom and brother, head tilted down, hands folded, I said this line and did a review of my week. Who had I hurt? Who did I need to apologize to? Who had hurt me? Who did I need to forgive?

Every Sunday my slate was wiped clean. God forgave me. Jesus forgave me (but then, I always thought of him as pretty easygoing; he forgave everything). Sure, I had to follow up by apologizing for hogging the slide at recess or forgetting (on purpose) to return a friend's Belinda Carlisle tape. I had to try to do better. But as I forgave, I was forgiven. I apologized for shoving my brother, and he and God forgave me. I got to start again. On the rare Sundays we weren't in church, I knelt on my bedroom floor and said the Lord's Prayer, feeling released from the weight of the world. I forgave those who had debted against me. God forgave me. I made up with friends. No debt went more than seven days. Reinforced on Sunday after Sunday was the healing notion that I was forgivable and had the power to forgive other people as well. No sin stained my soul permanently.

We human beings need rituals of forgiveness. I don't mean that we need to go to a church where we are berated about the sinfulness of our very existence, the so-called stain of our sexuality, our inherent badness—I don't believe in any of that. We are born with a clean slate and throughout our lives, despite good intentions, we sometimes mess up. We are selfish, petty, or mean. We pick on our siblings because we don't know how to say, "I need help." This doesn't make us inherently bad, soiled by sin, or in need of saving. But we do need ways to ask for, and receive, forgiveness. To release guilt and begin again.

In my Unitarian Universalist congregation, we share a Litany of Atonement created by Rev. Rob Eller-Isaacs. It begins,

> *For remaining silent, when a single voice would*
> *have made a difference,*
> *We forgive ourselves and each other; we begin*
> *again in love.*
> *For each time that our fears have made us*
> *rigid and inaccessible,*
> *We forgive ourselves and each other; we begin*
> *again in love.*
> *For each time that we have struck out in*
> *anger without just cause,*
> *We forgive ourselves and each other; we begin*
> *again in love.*

In my congregation we sing that last line, "We forgive ourselves and each other, we begin again in love." The music is chantlike and haunting, and as I bumble through my week, accidentally acting in fear instead of love, I hear the refrain in my head. We forgive ourselves. We forgive each other. We start again. And again. And again. A million times forgiven. Never permanently broken.

It's been many years since I scored my arms and legs with my fingernails, trying to release the hot burden of shame stuck in my body. It was my daily ritual for so long.

I no longer chant "stupid and mean" under my breath all day at school, in response to terrible grades and guilt at my cruelty toward my brother. I am not Lex Luthor or Judas or Stalin in pink footie pajamas. I forgive and I am forgiven. I am holy and human, and I get to begin again, in love.

7.

Mad Dog the Angry Adolescent

NONNI WAS LOUD, the loudest woman I knew. She screamed from the sidelines at our soccer matches, twice as loud as the dads, four times as loud as the other moms. With bleached blonde hair with a few inches of black roots, bright red lipstick, and painted-on black eyebrows, Nonni seemed to lack the self-consciousness of other women.

Nonni was Kirk's mom. Kirk was an adult, but he played on our middle school team because he had Down's syndrome. Nonverbal but communicative, Kirk would touch my arm comfortingly after a missed goal, his big brown eyes telegraphing empathy. Every kid in the league loved Kirk because he waved his arms happily in the air after either team scored, high-fiving kids on both sides. Kirk's dad was sweet but diminutive, silent but smiling. Nonni was tough enough for the three of them, her advocacy the reason Kirk got to play in a kid's league. Nonni was a powerful force. I heard other parents agree that she was "too much," and I found myself simultaneously fascinated and repulsed by her. I wanted her commanding presence; I loved the way everyone listened when she spoke. But I also saw the stigma she faced for being unfeminine. The other moms didn't talk to her, nor did the dads. She didn't play by the gender rules. That left her an outcast.

I was in sixth grade and trying to figure out what it meant to be feminine. Being liked by boys had suddenly become my friends' number one priority, an obsession bigger than New Kids on the Block and Barbies combined. Out of nowhere, the guys in our neighborhood went from gross—they tried to set their farts on fire!—to people who my friends actually wanted to impress. It didn't make sense to me, this sudden shift. These scrawny, longed-for males still thought it was hilarious to wipe their boogers on each other. To me, they were the same immature dorks they had been in elementary school. But my female peers said they were dreamy—so handsome, so manly. Were we even talking about the same boys? I didn't get it. But not liking boys was babyish and I didn't want to be babyish, so I pretended to be boy-crazy too. I was like Jane Goodall studying the mating behavior of apes—I didn't understand why my friends liked boys, but I could mimic their behavior in trying to attract them.

How to behave in order to attract a boy was our main question. We scoured *Teen, YM,* and *Seventeen* magazine to find clues. Makeup, which most of us were not allowed to wear, was apparently essential. As was smiling a lot, but not talking, which was hard for me. Not roughhousing, not yelling. Boys liked soft, quiet girls. Girls with pale white skin and long, horsey ponytails. Girls who laughed at boys' jokes but didn't make jokes of their own. Girls who didn't get dirty exploring the woods or playing sports but loved to sit on the sidelines and cheer for the boys while they played. It felt like attracting a boy meant turning into one of the pictures in the fashion magazines we studied: silent, pretty, and clean. Unreal.

At church that year we had a new associate minister, Jacque, who was young and cool and wore jeans to youth group meetings. Jacque had brown skin and huge, black eyes that crinkled at the edges when she laughed, which was often. Her hair was black, glossy, and thick. Her hands were rough from riding horses, and her arms rippled with muscles. I found her mesmerizing, a whole new version of beautiful. Better than any silent Barbie doll. I wanted black eyes and muscular arms too. Preaching on Sunday morning or sitting on the floor with us in Sunday School, Jacque seemed powerful, intelligent, and fearless. I wanted to be near her, but even more, I wanted to be her. When she stood in the pulpit in her black robe and red stole, my cheeks flushed and my heart raced. I hung on every word. It seemed a whole new way of being female was possible, dangerous but conceivable. And my mentor was right in front of me.

Jacque was the first church authority to show an interest in my ideas. It was like having Wonder Women leave the TV screen in order to ask me about my day. If I told her I liked her sermon, she wanted to know what, specifically, I liked about it. Which hymns did I like, and why? She wanted to know what images I pictured when I thought about God. She wanted the whole congregation to think about what it meant to call God the Father. What about the feminine aspects of God? What about God the Mother? What did it do to women, and women's rights, to make God a male?

This made most people in the congregation pretty uncomfortable, me included. How could I picture God, if not as a man? Didn't the Bible call God a he? I knew from the pictures in my Sunday school handouts that God and Jesus were boys. Mary was a girl, but she was only famous for being Jesus' mom. How boring: she was famous for being obedient. But Jacque talked about the errors inherent in biblical translations—the Hebrew, Greek, and Aramaic words being squeezed into Latin, then German, then English. Their meanings shifted as they moved from one tongue to another. Jacque talked about how different the ancient Israelite culture was from our own culture, how differently women were treated then.

Jacque said that the Bible was a description of how people thought about God in that Israelite culture, so very long ago. She blew all of our minds by talking about the Bible as a library of stories created by humans, men specifically. Stories that described how those particular men, with all of their biases, experienced God. Shockingly, the Bible wasn't written by God. It wasn't handed down by angels. It was an imperfect anthology of stories that often contradicted themselves. Jacque asked if we had noticed the multiple creation stories in Genesis or the differing directions Jesus gave to his disciples. I certainly hadn't noticed. The Bible had never been something to think about critically; it contained the instructions God gave to humans for how to live. Arguing with it would be like debating whether the grass should grow—it just did. The Bible just was the authority. But Jacque was showing us that it was much more complicated than that. That the Bible was one voice in a dialogue, with every believer taking the other voice. We got to debate the Bible, look at it in its cultural context, even disagree with it.

It is hard to describe how life altering it was to think about the Bible as fallible and God as anything other than an adult male. The notion that God was a man had colored every aspect of my life. Men were holy, women were not. Men were moral authorities, women were not. It was reflected in the incredible amount of attention my friends were focusing on attracting a male. Men were special, like gods. They were the main subject of our life stories, and we were side characters—girlfriends, wives, mothers. The holiness of men was reflected in my own family, where we tiptoed around my dad's temper. No one else was allowed to get so mad; no one else could have a temper tantrum. But Dad was special: he was the father. Like our God. Like Jesus when turning over tables in the temple, or God raging over the golden calf, men could be angry because their anger was sacred.

As my theology evolved, my body entered puberty. My hips pushed outward and my waist in. My breasts grew obvious enough that my parents insisted I start wearing a bra. I started to menstruate. The whole thing seemed like a big hassle, another thing to deal with that my brother didn't have to. The binding feeling of the bra, stiff wires digging into my young skin; the bulky sanitary pads, period cramps. There wasn't anything fun about the added burdens of puberty. Still, I didn't think about it much until men started to act weird around me, strangers looking at my chest or making remarks in passing.

Unwelcome attention from men became a big problem. Latchkey kids in the summer, my brother and I spent our days riding to the neighborhood pool on our bicycles or exploring the woods pretending to be Indiana Jones. Lately, men in pickup trucks had started slowing down to yell at me as I rode, leering at me in my swimsuit and old cut-off jeans. Their harassment caused a welling up of hot shame and raw panic in my chest. It made me want to get inside my house and stay there. I didn't want their eyes or hands to find me, to catch me. My new breasts made me into prey. Predators were everywhere.

At the first day of soccer practices that fall, my coach, a local college student, looked me up and down for a long time, finally saying, "Well, someone certainly grew up over the summer." It made my skin crawl, this man-sized beast sliding his eyes over my new breasts and hips. I felt like I had done something wrong to get this kind of attention from a grown-up. Before that year, I doubt he could remember my name. Now he noticed me, at every game putting a hand on my shoulder or waist—nothing illegal, but still much more attention than I'd garnered when I had the body of a little girl.

I knew the textbook basics of hetero sex: a man and a woman love each other very much, they get married and want to make a baby, penis in vagina, baby comes nine months later. I knew that sometimes, shockingly, marriage wasn't even involved. But what did any of that have to do with me? I still played with dolls, with a Ouija board at sleepovers. I didn't have sexual urges. Why were grown men hollering at me? What had changed? I had never seen pornography or even a sexy scene in a movie. I truly couldn't imagine what these men wanted.

Around that time, conversations about virginity and purity pacts began to take over girls' conversations in the school lunchroom. While most of my friends were Christians, I was beginning to see how much diversity fit under that title. My closest friend, Nadine, was a hardcore born-again. She talked about the Blood of the Lamb in casual conversation and regularly cried for all the aborted babies. She told us to be on our best behavior because Jesus was coming any second. Nadine believed in absolutely no sexual contact before marriage—not even French kissing (which sounded totally gross anyway). She said virginity was like a piece of chewing gum—no one wanted to chew prechewed gum. Likewise, no man wanted to marry a woman who had already had sex.

Nadine admitted that the rules for men were different, but that was because males are weak. She said the devil can move in a girl to make her tempt a boy. And once boys start getting excited, they cannot stop until their lust is relieved; it's "biological science," she claimed. It's not their fault if they push things too far. So no getting boys excited with low-cut shirts or short-shorts. Nadine had a purity ring, a fancy emerald and gold confection, that her father gave her when she turned twelve. The ring was her promise to remain pure for her future husband—meaning no sex or sexy activity—and then return the ring to her dad on the altar when he delivered her to her groom, where she would swap it for a wedding ring.

It freaked me out, the idea of talking to my dad so openly about sex. I didn't even like asking him to buy me period pads. But Shannon, who was Christian but didn't go to church except on Christmas Eve, said God had bigger problems than worrying about virginity. Besides, if you waited to have sex until you were married, how would you know if the sex was any good? How would you know if your husband was doing it right? Shannon's mom went on lots of dates and said there was a huge difference between men who knew how to do it and men who didn't. What if you married a dud? Better to sleep with a few guys before settling down so you knew you got a good sex partner. Shannon said she had promised her mom not to have sex until she was sixteen because doing it before then would make people think she was slutty. Then she planned to have sex with five guys before getting married. The group agreed that five sex partners seemed like enough to get an idea of what to expect, enough to know what was good and not good before committing. All except Nadine, who started praying out loud that Shannon be saved before she had a chance to have premarital sex and be thrown into the fiery pit of Hell. Then Nadine and Shannon started arguing about whether Shannon was a real Christian, debating baptism, confession, and piety in a way I wouldn't be familiar with until seminary.

Around that time, Jacque decided that our youth group needed to talk about sex. This was, unfortunately, the same night as my parents volunteered to chaperone, so I spent the evening praying for the embarrassment to actually kill me. But I did pick up a few things. First, Jacque said sex was a pleasurable, romantic act. I hadn't heard that anywhere else. School sex ed was focused on anatomy and condoms:

what went in where and how to not get STIs. It was scientific and practical (for heterosexuals) but didn't go into when or why a person should have sex, and we certainly didn't bring God into it. It was mostly scary, with lots of pictures of private parts covered in rashes and warts.

Nadine thought sex was an awful thing that women had to do to get babies, and Shannon thought it was a fun thing to do that unfortunately sometimes led to babies. But Jacque said sex was a blessing because it feels good and bonds you with your partner. She said it was a gift from God—something God gave us because God loves us. An act to share with the person you love the most. Jacque said that she thought we should wait until we were married to have sex because sex is sacred, a holy thing to save for holy matrimony. But she admitted that most people didn't wait and that waiting might not feel practical. She said that was okay, that God wouldn't send us to Hell for it. Again, sex was a gift, with no strings. We got to choose how to enjoy it, as long as it was consensual and loving.

She suggested—and remember that Jacque was an American Baptist minister—that we learn to masturbate so we could cope with our sexual urges and learn what we liked. That way we wouldn't be overcome with horniness in the back of a car and end up having sex with someone we didn't love. Jacque said that sex bonds people together and if we had sex with someone we didn't care about or who didn't care about us, we might feel really sad and confused.

This was a tremendous amount of confusing information for me to take in. First, I wasn't yet into the horny stage of adolescents, being a late bloomer. The idea that horniness could take over a person's brain, like being possessed by a demon in a horror movie, sounded terrifying. The idea that I would find someone I loved enough to want to take my clothes off in front of and do all the weird things in the sex ed filmstrip seemed unlikely. I had previously thought that masturbating was just a gross thing boys did. Anything Jacque suggested was cool to me, but I didn't even know where to begin with masturbation.

I took my new, church-sanctioned information back to the school lunchroom. Everyone was shocked, but for different reasons. Nadine agreed that sex was special married-people activity but not that women could find it pleasurable. She definitely thought a woman went to Hell for premarital sex (but again, not men, because they are weak and God understands that). She thought Jacque was certainly not a real minister and was probably Satan in disguise—and that was before I told her about the encouragement to masturbate!

Shannon didn't see what was so special about sex. She heard her mom having sex all the time—was I saying there was something sinful about her mom? She also thought the masturbation thing was weird because masturbation was for guys and desperate women who were too ugly to get guys to have sex with them. Soon after this conversation,

Shannon got a boyfriend and joined the popular crowd. We smiled at each other in the hallways but understood that our worlds were now too different for us to be friends. Nadine talked to her mom about what I learned at youth group, and her mom talked to their preacher, who said she shouldn't socialize with me anymore except when she saw an opportunity to bring me to Christ. Nadine told me tearfully that she couldn't be my friend anymore, unless maybe I wanted to go to Bible camp with her?

It was a frustrating time of life. The girls like Shannon, who were anointed by having a boy pick them as a girlfriend, entered a kind of club the rest of us couldn't access. Boys decided who was popular, and the best friend alliances of elementary school disappeared. I was not one of the chosen girls. I frequently forgot to brush my hair. I was loud. I argued in class. I was good at debate, and I liked to do it—a quality that was seemingly a good thing until adolescence, when suddenly girls were supposed to be nice and not show boys up, not make them feel bad at any cost. This was one of many new middle school rules that everyone seemed to know but that I was just starting to figure out.

My love of the science fair, while always nerdy, was now also suspect—science fair was for boys. Riding your bike to the pool to actually swim or roughhouse in the water was for babies and boys. The cool adolescent girls walked to the pool—a bike helmet would muss their hair. They lounged by the water and looked pretty; they were available for boys to talk to when they got out of the water. I didn't understand why fun seemed to be uncool now. Why was being looked at better than being active? Why would I want to watch boys have fun instead of having fun myself?

I was frustrated with no outlet—my friends had all gone over to the boy-crazy side. Home was tense, with my dad under the family curse—happy one moment and furious the next. The cat had chewed the face off of one of my dolls, and I had unwittingly imitated him by screaming, "God damn it, Fluffy, what the hell is wrong with you?" This provoked stunned laughter and then fury from my parents, with my dad yelling, "Where the hell did you learn to swear?" with no sense of irony.

My mom had begun to restrict my movement for reasons I didn't understand, but which had to do with the men honking at me in my swimsuit and with Jacque's sex talk. No more exploring the woods alone, no more riding my bike home after dark. I was getting older, so why was I allowed fewer freedoms? And why didn't my brother, two years younger, have to follow any of those rules? It made me resent my body and want to be a little kid again. Growing up didn't seem to have any advantages.

Which takes me back to Nonni at the soccer field, loud Nonni yelling on the sidelines. I didn't have any healthy outlets for my anger, so soccer became where I expressed rage. That year, I transformed from a not-really-interested soccer player into an aggressive one, and Nonni was the first to notice. I was pissed at being made into a sexual object. I was furious that the rules had changed and that appealing to boys was now the priority. I missed Nadine and Shannon. Being a preteen sucked.

Moreover, I was mad at God and my church. Jacque had opened my eyes to the danger of thinking of God as a man, and now I saw the negative repercussions of that male worship all around me. Men had created God in their image, and women were just objects to be leered at, to look pretty and be quiet. Why had God allowed it? Why had I spent the first decade of my life worshiping God the Father? Why had my church taught me to worship the idea of a male God? So many adults at church, people I loved and who loved me, were furious at Jacque for bringing the truth to us that God is bigger than one gender. But Jacque had made a bigger, more complete God visible to me. Why did my church family resent her for it? I was furious—about puberty, about my involuntary objectification, and about my perfect church family not being so perfect after all.

I got on the soccer field and let the ball, and the shins of my fellow players, feel the brunt of my rage. I charged players much larger than me, boys who had hit early growth spurts and ran like colts on the field, unwieldy legs lurching unpredictably under them. Furious at the world, I ran right into them, throwing them off balance. I kicked them in the shins, I stepped on their feet, I tripped them—and I was never called on a foul. The boys often were, but the referees just couldn't believe that a petite little girl like me could be the aggressor. "Those boys were playing too rough!" the refs said, pointing them off the field.

But Nonni saw through my shenanigans. She knew what I was up to, and she loved it. Maybe she remembered her own adolescent rage; maybe she recognized me as a future fellow feminist—but she would yell, "Go, Kate! Get in there, Mad Dog—show 'em how it's done! Give 'em hell, Mad Dog!"

For a sixth-grade girl, the nickname Mad Dog was a social nightmare. Before the week was out, I was called that on the bus and in the school hallways. I hated it, but it was accurate. I was enraged and, like a powerless pet, had no socially acceptable way to vent that anger, so I turned to violence. On the soccer field, I expelled my anger by being mean, by being the opposite of what was expected for a girl. I battered and bruised the boys I played against as a big "screw that" to the idea that I should be pretty and quiet. And soon my coach stopped looking at me lasciviously and instead stayed away from me, seemingly nervous in my presence.

Now I am proud of my nickname, Mad Dog, even if I'm not proud that I took out my anger on the shins and feet of boys who were in their own adolescent hell. They didn't invent the patriarchy. And with or without the nickname Mad Dog, my social status was bound to plummet that year, as girls and boys punished me for not fulfilling my gender's prescribed role. I was the lowest of the low in terms of popularity, but in retrospect that was a good place to be. Other girls in the social-reject caste still played with dolls, rode bikes, and roughhoused at the pool. None of us had any hope of attracting a boyfriend, so we didn't spend much time worrying about it. Being unpopular gave us the space to continue figuring out who we were and what we liked without the pressure to conform that the cool girls faced.

It is disgusting that grown men treated me—at age ten!—as a sexual object. What the hell was my soccer coach, twice my age, thinking when he licked his lips while looking me over? I wish I could simultaneously empower and protect the girls that I know, shielding them from the harmful intentions of predators while encouraging them to explore the woods and ride their bikes after dark. Tell them there is more to life than being the object of some boy's or man's desire. But it's hard when women are so routinely discounted for not being attractive enough, for being too loud or too shrill. Who can forget the 2016 presidential election? Clinton was criticized for her clothes, her wrinkles, for looking tired. . . . At the Clinton/Trump debates, she walked a fine line in calling Trump out on blatant lies while trying to be feminine and nice at the same time. She could never raise her voice. And Clinton is a white woman! Consider that a Black woman can't raise her voice without being seen as angry and therefore dangerous. Consider that Latina women can't be angry without being called crazy. There is no socially acceptable way to be a powerful, independent woman, especially for a woman of color.

With all the pressure on girls and women to be passive but attractive, calm, and quiet, isn't it a wonder that we aren't all kicking men in the shins, knocking them over, stepping on their feet? The self-control of women is immeasurably powerful. Perhaps Nonni recognized in me a fellow Mad Dog, raging against a world brutally unfair to girls and women. Can we channel that rage, that self-control, into creativity, building a world in which girls are not prey but adventurers, scientists, and explorers? Free to ride bikes after dark, roughhouse in the pool, and tear through the woods, figuring out who they are? I want girls to stop being objects to be admired and start being the subjects of their own stories.

True equality cannot come until we dismantle the idea that God is male. Jacque pushed my church family to evolve in ways that we initially found incredibly uncomfortable—it hurts when we challenge ideas that are precious to us. But ultimately, we discovered a bigger, bolder, more diverse God. A God unchained by patriarchal ideas about who gets to be powerful and who gets to judge. She pushed our youth group to talk about sex in a way far from the shame-based rhetoric of conservative religion but still just as holy. It was radical on both fronts: sex positive and still guided by sacred values.

Every girl needs role models like Nonni, who can seem like "too much" while being exactly what a girl needs. Like Jacque, who took an idea so dear to me—God the Father—

and helped me to expand it to a God much bigger than one gender, one metaphor, one being. Who told me sex wasn't dirty or casual but sacred and fun. Who told me to explore my own body without shame. Girls need to know women who aren't passive and quiet, women with rough hands and red lipstick, women who refuse to sit on the sidelines and watch the boys. Thank God for loud, powerful women.

8.

Technicolor Romance

I MET DREW for the first time on a technicolor dream of a late-summer day. It was our first year of college, and freshman orientation was in full swing. My college isn't for supersmart kids; it isn't prestigious or elite. But it does get all the extra points for being idyllic. It looks like a college straight from central casting: a red brick and fresh white paint campus tucked into the rolling foothills of the Appalachians, with a silver lake in the center complete with wandering geese. Verdant trees shaded young scholars and hung-over frat guys from the bright Ohio sun. Professors and students conversed on long, closely clipped lawns. The sky was robin's egg blue; the leaves were emerald green. The air, thick with birdsong, smelled of fresh-cut hay and wildflowers. It looked just like college was supposed to look, as different from the strip malls and billboards of home as possible. The fresh breezes brought the scent of cornfields instead of the Cargill corn-processing plant that I grew up smelling. At night, the only sounds were crickets and frogs. It was paradise.

I chose my college for a simple reason: it was the college that accepted me. I made dismal grades throughout high school, so I was lucky to get in anywhere. In my first days on campus, I was afraid this historic institution would realize their error, and some sort of academic guard would come pull me out of the classroom—a Robocop in academic robes, the *Complete Works of Heidegger* tucked under his arm as he hurried me off campus. But as the days passed, I relaxed. I lounged on manicured lawns, munched apples nicked from the dining hall while strolling under the maple trees on the way to class.

I was in the dining hall, a cacophonous space full of undergrads, sitting with new friends. We were talking about our "type," the kinds of guys we were into. Looking around, we saw muscly guys sporting shirts from their high school football team, guys with unironic plastic glasses talking about Dungeons and Dragons, guys with cool plastic glasses talking about bands, frat guys with beer bellies, and hippie guys with hemp chokers, talking about where to score weed. Sensitive guys self-consciously reading poetry alone, looking moody. None of these guys were my type. And then Drew walked in.

Drew was a deep nut brown from a summer in the sun. He had eyes of sea-glass green and long, curly hair that skimmed his muscular shoulders. He looked like an Italian version of Pearl Jam's Eddie Veder. I was in lust at first sight. He also had on an embarrassingly unironic t-shirt, one of those inspirational slogan shirts that says "Drive Is the Difference Between Winners and Losers" and has a picture of a snake eating a cheetah or something. He was perfect in his imperfection. I had to find a way to meet him.

The next day, all the first-year students were gathered on the quad for corny ice-breaking games, and I made sure to end up next to Drew. I was funny and kept tossing my hair over my shoulder, which I thought guys liked but probably just seemed weirdly compulsive. I laughed a lot and made aggressive eye contact. Still, it took a few months of us awkwardly flirting before we started dating.

I had boyfriends in high school, sweet guys who played Beatles songs on their acoustic guitars and could talk about their feelings. We were much more "friends who made out" than in love. They were the kinds of guys I would be happy for my niece to date—earnest, well meaning, and naïve. After the relationship ended, we were always friends. But dating in college had an edge of danger that I felt both drawn to and repelled by. I was far from home and living in a dorm, so my parents weren't going to suddenly come home and interrupt any physical romance. That was both scary and thrilling. And the guys were more of a mystery.

Back home, my parents knew the parents of my boyfriends. Often we had grown up together, played on the same t-ball team as third graders. There were no surprises. Everyone knew everyone. But these guys were from other cities, some even from other states. They might as well have been from another planet. It was so hot.

In retrospect, Drew wasn't so different from all my earlier boyfriends. He was shy, artistic, and kind. He always walked me back to my dorm after campus events and would tuck my hand inside his glove, our fingers ensconced in wool together. He wrote me poetry and brought flowers when I was in school productions. When I was too sick with the flu to go to the dining hall, he snuck me out an entire Boston cream pie. When I told him I was a feminist, he said, "Me too—or my mom is, so I guess I am. That's how that works, right?" I told him feminism was about equality, not birthright, and he assured me that he was pro-equality. Drew was a progressive Christian, raised in an open-minded Catholic family. He loved God. He wanted to serve the world somehow.

There was nothing dangerous about Drew, but I fell in love anyway. Having a dad with anger management problems makes calm, quiet men incredibly sexy to me. I have millions of fond memories of our four years in college together, even though my final year we trudged through hell together.

I entered my senior year ready to put a sweet cherry on top of the hot fudge sundae that was college. I was sharing a big, old, yellow house off campus with five friends and taking fairly easy classes. Having just returned from a semester abroad, I was ready to wow everyone with my Sabrina-like European transformation (which was really just me with shorter hair and wearing red lipstick). I wanted to move to New York City after graduation, or Paris, or heck, Chicago—it didn't matter, I just wanted an adventure. Applications for internships all over the world were piled on my desk.

I had a rough start with my housemates. We had all been friends for a few years, but second-string friends. People I was friendly with, but we didn't go out together. We ate together in the cafeteria, but I didn't call them on the phone. I had forgotten about finding a roommate before I left for Europe, and by the time I remembered, it was live with these friends or live in the dorms. Perish the thought! Besides, these were cool women, feminist women. I knew them all from campus chapel services.

However, they were more conservative than I had anticipated. It was church camp all over again. I knew they were Christian but figured they were religious like me—liberal do-gooders who think gay folks are great and abortion is a human right. I was way off. They hung Jesus posters in the living room and tried to declare the house a no-alcohol zone. No alcohol? I had just returned from England, where having a pint in your local pub was a social responsibility. It was your duty, your contribution to upholding English culture and creating communal bonds (or so I told my parents). But my roomies were saying no booze, no parties, no guys on the second floor. . . . Was this a nunnery?

But we were sorting it out. I convinced them that drinking wine was sophisticated, not like drinking keg beer. Jesus turned water into wine! It was classy. I brought home a few jugs of super-sweet, super-cheap red wine and served it with cheese and baguettes, and soon the no-booze rule was overturned in order to institute Wine Wednesdays. I was still working on the no-parties rule. Parties didn't have to mean debauchery (unless they were really good parties). But we bonded and quickly became good friends.

A few weeks into the quarter, I realized I'd had the same nervous stomachache for a few days. Then I started getting headaches. I wasn't sleeping well. Anxiety wasn't new to me; I was always a nervous person. But my college years had been a respite. I was more relaxed and confident than at any other time of my life. I was able to learn in class because my mind wasn't tied up with worry. I could focus on big projects and memorize my lines for plays. The Kate who barely passed classes seemed far in the past—I was a straight-A student with big parts in college plays, a work-study job building sets for those plays, lots of friends, and a sweet boyfriend. Why was my childhood anxiety back to bother me? My life was going so well.

You know that moment in a horror film when you're sure the heroine is going to die? She trips in the woods when the bad guy is right behind her, and although she has survived close calls before, this time she isn't going to be so lucky. One day, that awful certainty hit me as I was walking to class. I was terrified and that utter terror was spiked with deep, bottomless hopelessness. It was a two-block walk on a gorgeous fall day to a class I liked. Gold and orange leaves were gently falling, and the sun was bright in the sapphire sky. But I couldn't take a deep breath. I gasped ineffectually. My heart pumped with a wild out-of-control abandon. I wanted to run away from an invisible monster; I felt the end of my life was near. My stomach churned painfully. But as I scanned the street for some threat, some danger to make sense of my body's sudden propulsion into terror, I saw that there was no predator.

This made the wide maw of hopelessness grow until I was tumbling into its pit, weeping at my fate, because surely these sensations meant I was going to die. What was wrong with my body? If there was no external threat, there must be one inside of me. A heart attack, an aneurysm—heck, I would have believed I had Ebola. Something in my body had ruptured, and soon I would be dead. I cried from fear—surely it would be painful, this approaching death—and sorrow. I wasn't ready to leave this world. I ran home, crying for my family, for Drew, for my friends, all the souls I loved but would not see again. Wracked with grief, I fell onto my bed, sobbing for an hour or so before I fell asleep—not calm, but physically exhausted from the coursing adrenaline in my body.

People think anxiety is "all in your head," as if a good self-talking-to would discipline it out of your life. But panic disorder manifests all over the body. Remember learning about fight or flight? Anxiety attacks make the heart race—mine beats like I've run a marathon sometimes when I'm just sitting on my couch. My breath shortens and my chest constricts. This signals my body to shunt all my blood to my vital organs, so my hands and feet get cold and tingly. I start to feel lightheaded as blood courses south. My stomach flips and flops and I feel nauseous, and sometimes I dry heave or throw up stomach acid. I'm not sure how to explain what happens to my legs except that they want to run. They feel like they need to run as fast and hard as possible. Walking or running up steep hills is the only thing that relieves them, and the relief only lasts while I am still moving.

Now I have coping strategies, a banal phrase meaning I have tricks to abate the feelings of utter terror and grief. I take deep breaths from the lowest part of my stomach: inhaling as slowly as possible, pausing while my body is absolutely stuffed with air, and exhaling slowly. I move my body, getting outside if I can, putting my hands on trees and trying to focus on the texture of their trunks. I run up and down flights of stairs. I listen to classical or New Age music, the annoying kind with chimes and singing bowls. I do push-ups, which I really hate—if I'm doing push-ups, things are really rough. I take a very hot and then very cold shower; I pop a prescription sedative and find a calming meditation video online. I also take a daily antianxiety pill that seems to put a cap on how bad things can get.

I didn't have coping skills in college. The day I was terrified of going to class I longed for a deep gulp of wine, but I'm glad that I didn't have any in the house. Lots and lots of people self-medicate anxiety disorder with alcohol; any AA meeting is stuffed with stories about undiagnosed panic disorder. I drink alcohol with friends, socially, but I'm careful about not drinking to medicate my mental illness. When I'm anxious, I order soda. Booze would numb the awful feelings in the moment, but the addiction isn't worth it.

My great-uncle John, my mom's uncle, came home from World War I traumatized by all he saw in Japan. He had endless nightmares and panic attacks; he cried and shook. At the time, the treatment for posttraumatic stress disorder was to tell young men to toughen up and get busy doing whatever would distract them. This technique didn't do anything except make vets who couldn't just "buck up" feel like failures. Uncle John was one of few men in my family who wasn't a teetotaler—not after the war anyway. Without medication for his fits of utter terror, he turned to alcohol. Uncle John lost his wife, his job, and his independent adult life to alcoholism, but with no medical alternative, it was probably still better than a life of daily panic and war flashbacks.

I didn't tell my friends or even Drew about my panic attack. I didn't know what to call it, how to even begin to explain what had happened. I wasn't embarrassed, but how could I describe it? It didn't make any sense. I pushed it from my mind and continued like life was normal. But every day I felt a little worse. I felt scared, like I had when I was worried about my dad's temper but turned up a thousand notches. And there was nothing to be scared about. It made me feel crazy. Soon it was time to go home for a week for Thanksgiving break. I hoped that sleeping in and eating home cooking would force the weird feelings to abate. But a few days in, my mom asked what I was hoping to do after graduation, and I immediately started crying and shaking. I couldn't imagine moving to New York or Paris or Chicago with the painful fear that had recently taken over my body. All of my postgraduation hopes felt impossible. I think my mom recognized immediately that I had Dad's panic disorder, and she called him downstairs.

I would love to explain why I didn't immediately realize that I was having an anxiety attack, just like my dad, and get some help. I really don't know why I didn't see that I had what he had. But I wasn't yelling; I just felt afraid. There was no rage; rage seemed like a powerful feeling, and I felt weak and helpless. During most of my childhood, I had felt a lesser version of this—nervous stomach, lightheadedness, racing heart—but I never thought it was mental illness. It was just a bizarre thing about me that I didn't talk about.

My parents took me to the family doctor, who assured me that she had pills that would help and that I would be back to normal in a month or so. Which for most people would probably have been true, but those pills didn't work. When it was time to head back to campus, I stayed home, still having anxiety attacks and crying more and more regularly. My mind was sick of being nervous and was giving in to despair. This is a normal phenomenon for women with untreated depression—the fear turns to hopelessness. In men, the fear turns into rage. Either way, it is intensely painful.

My second round of pills didn't work, so then I got to go to a psychiatrist, a jolly old man with marionettes decorating his office, who assured me he could crack my anxiety with a new combination of pills. When I came back a few weeks later, weeping, he told me to stop the theatrics—he had trouble believing I felt as awful as I described. I felt like I was ruining his fun—he wanted to be the hero who cured me, and I was spoiling that by not getting better. I spent a lot of time and energy trying to tell him that I was entering a new phase of my disorder. I was fantasizing about suicide and it felt terrifying, but as I tried prescription after prescription without any relief, it started to feel inevitable.

Meanwhile, Drew was back at our idyllic college, trying to dodge questions about where I was. Mental illness was still stigmatized at our small institution, where everyone knew everyone and gossip flew through the halls. He told only my closest friends and called me every night. He was baffled by my panic attacks; he had only known me as a happy, successful college student. He researched anxiety disorders and visited as often as his roommate would loan him his car. He never lost hope that I would recover. I couldn't tell him about my suicidal fantasies. I couldn't tell anyone except for my overly cheerful psychologist, who didn't believe me anyway.

9.

Psych Hospital, Version One

THE HOSPITAL WALLS were an odd, uneven yellow, more the dingy shade of white stained by cigarette smoke than the forcefully cheerful Buttercup or Sunbeam of a can of paint. There was an elongated bedpan tacked to the wall in the place of a mirror and no rope pulls on the drapes—no chance to commit suicide here. I noted these things in my Xanax- and sleep-clouded mind before I heard the inhuman groans of my roommate—noises like a bear caught in a trap, agony and grief mixed with weariness. Sounds that implied a question: how much more could she take?

I rolled over to look at her as she began a stream of grumbles that became a scream. "No no no no—give it to me give it to me! Give it to me give it to me give it to me—" I didn't know what she wanted but felt her cries were urgent enough to warrant my going for help, so I slid from between the sheets and padded on the cold linoleum to the hallway.

Late the night before, when I'd been admitted to the psych ward, the space was quiet. Earlier that night, after dinner, I had told my parents that I couldn't quit thinking about all the pills in the medicine cabinet—I couldn't quit thinking about gulping every bottle. Again and again, I imagined the feeling of the pills tumbling down my throat, handful after handful. How quiet it would then become. Then I could swim out past the tidal waves of misery that crashed into me all day. I imagined it would be like the peace of sleeping without the inevitable waking in the morning. Mornings were the worst time of day—opening my eyes and realizing I had to suffer through another day in the sea of agony. The handfuls of pills would bring stillness without waking.

But a small, persistent part of me believed that I could get better, that life could get back to normal. That someday I might be happy again, in some mysterious future time. A tiny part of me remembered that just months before, I had laughed until my stomach hurt, feeling real joy unaided by pharmaceuticals. Like a book I had enjoyed but now could only remember the feeling of, memories of happiness lurked at one corner of my vision. And that slip of a memory sent me downstairs to confess my suicidal fantasies.

My dad called a behavioral health hotline provided by his health insurance company and an eerily calm therapist said to take me to the emergency room. I didn't want to be hospitalized, but I wasn't getting better seeing my psychiatrist every other week. None of the myriad of soothing-sounding pills had snapped me out of my agony, and I didn't think my doctor realized how utterly hopeless I felt. Maybe the hospital would. Maybe the doctors there would have a magical pill my psychiatrist didn't know about.

The three of us walked into the ER, a parent on each side of me, holding each of my arms, as if my problem was a sprained ankle instead of a broken psyche. The sleepy nurse at intake barked, "What is your emergency?," and my mom answered, "We are feeling kind of suicidal tonight."

"All of you?" she replied unsympathetically. My mom said, "No, just Kate." We were assigned a room where we waited a few hours to meet a social worker. I commenced my regular evening routine of hysterical crying fragmented by brief stints of unsatisfying sleep. Then I was admitted, given a large enough dose of some sedative to have to be put in a wheelchair, and carted up to the psych ward.

Now morning had arrived, and I was in the hallway trying to flag down a nurse, afraid that my roommate was dying. The sedative made me cloudy enough to hug the walls as I walked, intoxicated but determined. Finally, I spotted the nurse's station and stumbled in that direction, realizing I had only a hospital gown on as I felt a chill on my backside. Great—I was in a brightly lit hallway, surrounded by strangers, with only a fairly transparent shirt on that was open at the back, and no undies. Friends bragged about streaking the college quad—did this count? Could I claim this while playing the drinking game "Never Have I Ever"—never have I ever streaked a psych ward hallway while trying to save my possibly dying roommate?

I reached the counter without incident, and the nurse looked at me over her reading glasses: "Roommate trouble?" I related that I was pretty sure she was dying and the nurse mumbled, "She feels like it, anyway," and told me to sit in the common room while they checked on her. I went back to put on clothes—no more nudie time for me— and as I dug in the drawers in the dark room, my roommate stopped moaning for a moment and asked, "You ever done heroin?" I shook my head. "Don't—it's a bitch to get out of your system." I thanked her for the advice and scrambled out of the room. She resumed screeching like she was giving birth to an elephant.

Did you know that at small hospitals the drug detox space is in the psych ward? So people with panic disorders— people who hear voices, people who can't escape crushing feelings of sadness, people who doubt their own reality— can be paired with people going through excruciating withdrawal. It reminded me of my dad's old joke: I would go to him with a headache and he would lightly pinch my arm and say, "And now your arm hurts. Does that take your mind off your headache?" If we psych patients thought we had it bad, we could check out how awful detoxing feels! Hey kids, don't take drugs!

Still in a Xanax fog, I wandered into the common room where a TV was blaring *Good Morning America*. It seemed criminal for anyone to be as perky as the blonde hostess talking about a dog beauty pageant like it was a vital news story. Thinking violent thoughts about her, I turned to a half-finished puzzle of an English cottage bedecked in flowers. There were half a dozen pieces left on the table, the puzzle clearly requiring dozens more to be completed. There was a man begging a chair for help in the corner—another detoxer, or perhaps a schizophrenic? I quickly reversed course to a pile of worn *National Geographic* magazines by a threadbare, plastic-covered couch (how did it get so worn out with the plastic over it? Did they wait for it to look like damp garbage before they put down a protective cover?) and grabbed a publication at least twenty years old. Flipping it open to a random page, I started to relax—just in time for a filthy man of forty or seventy to slide up next to me, much too close. He smelled like the couch looked, all rotten teeth and the aroma of dried sweat and dirty clothes.

"You like that, do you? Me too. Maybe we can get together and look at those pictures privately. Be educational." He leered at me and then at the *National Geographic*, which had fallen open to a full-page picture of a topless woman breastfeeding in some faraway land. Before

I could wheel back and either smack him, vomit, or both, a woman's voice rang out from across the room. "Mel, you leave her alone. She's a fancy girl, look at her. Probably had braces, rode a horse, some shit like that. She doesn't need you bothering her."

Mel shot a stream of curse words in her direction but got up and left me alone, to my great relief. I smiled at her and she quickly asked, "Got a cigarette? Got anyone who will bring you cigarettes? Weed? You got cash?" At the shake of my head, she replied, "Fine, you'll find some way to pay me back later."

Five minutes in the common room and I had been propositioned and now owed a strange woman a favor. Awesome. I learned pretty quickly that any favor had to be repaid—ideally in cigarettes, but giving them your dessert worked in a pinch. I also learned that being white, having all my teeth, and wearing clean clothes that were mine, and not from the free closet the social worker administered, would quickly get me labeled a snob and full of myself. When word got around that the rich white girl didn't have access to tobacco products and wasn't fooling around with anyone sexually, people lost interest in me fast. Which was fine—I didn't come to the psych ward to make lifelong friends. But it was awkward to decide where to sit at meals, like the high school cafeteria all over again.

Should I sit with the postnatal depression moms, whose family members brought their tiny babies in every few hours so they could breastfeed? They cried all the time, like me, but were five or ten years older. I could sit with the drug-detoxing teenagers, who were my age, but the detoxers stayed away from the mental health patients—as one teen girl said during group therapy, "At least I'm crazy because of drugs. They were just born nuts." There were class and race rules to navigate. Black people sat with Black people, white people with white people, and since there wasn't a quorum of any other minority, the few Latinx and Asian folks sat alone. Folks living on the street sat together, with foster kids at the far end of their table. White people from the burbs took up a table by the door, closest to the food and bathrooms, asserting dominance consciously or subconsciously.

If you were disruptive enough—yelled at things no one else could see, took off your clothes at inopportune times—you got to eat in your room. I was too much of a good girl to act out just to get privacy while eating, so I rushed to get to the dining room first so I could sit down at an empty table and not risk offending anyone by sitting in the wrong spot. I grabbed a spot in the corner and read the old *National Geographic*s during the meal, carefully avoiding any pages with nudity. And I cried, which was not unusual or noteworthy in the psych ward.

Between meals, we were kept busy with group therapy in the morning and occupational therapy in the afternoon. In group therapy, a psychotherapist prodded us to consider our coping skills: how we managed the difficulties of every-day life. Which is helpful to consider, but we were in too big and diverse a group for it to be useful for us to talk about together. The problems we faced were so different: a woman who kept getting kicked out of homeless shelters because she responded to the voices in her mind. A young man strug-gling to detox and stay off heroin while living with his mom who used drugs multiple times a day and didn't like that he was trying to quit because then he might think he was better than her. Moms with incredible guilt over being away from their babies while getting treatment for postnatal depres-sion. Our situations were all different, but our goal was the same: to not end our lives. Staying alive in the waves of despair. Not giving up.

In the afternoon, we made birdhouses with the occupa-tional therapist. I don't remember why, just that I cried while trying to nail the pieces together and then cried more when I realized I had done it wrong and had to pull the tiny nails back out. I hit my finger with the hammer, but since I was already crying, no one noticed. I kept thinking, "bird houses for the birdbrains" and giggling, earning me con-cerned looks from the therapist.

All this happened while I was in a drug-induced daze. I was trying out different combinations of medications, the doctors trying to halt, or at least slow down, the waves of sadness. They felt that if they could just get a small break in the misery, a brief respite, that psychotherapy and a few good pharmaceuticals could get me back on track. But so far, the pills had been ineffective. So they added more medications, and I swallowed handfuls of pills, six or seven every day. Then they added medications to treat the side effects of the psych meds—a laxative, a sleep drug, and caffeine pill in the morning to burn off the sleeping pill.

The doctors were in a hurry. Insurance companies give patients about seven days, at the absolute maximum, to get better and get out of the hospital. That is almost always an impossible feat—psych meds take three or four weeks to start to be effective. So doctors try to guess what might work and discharge patients as soon as they promise they aren't going to commit suicide. This means there is a huge rate of patients being readmitted, often after just a few days. It also means a lot of patients feel a bit better in the security and stability of the hospital, then go home (or back to living on the street), feel awful again, and before the meds start working, they end their lives. Or they hold on until the meds are supposed to start working, but the combination the doctors chose doesn't work for them, and feeling like failures, like they will never recover, they end their lives.

It often takes months to find the right combination of medications. Doctors and pharmacologists don't really know why some drugs work on some people and others do not. In decades past, doctors kept psych patients in the hospital for six months at a time, trying medications out. They had talk therapy and learned relaxation techniques, did yoga, prayed with the chaplain, painted with watercolors. People learned to relax and had time to think about what was working in their lives and what wasn't. Time away from family and friends gave them time to evaluate those relationships. When patients left the hospital, they were on a drug regimen that has been successful for at least a month or two. They had new coping skills. People were able to take the time to get better. There was less suicide and much less going back to inpatient care.

It's hard to imagine how insurance companies justify kicking suicidal patients out of the hospital so quickly, often after just three days. Certainly, the stigma associated with mental illness is a part of this neglect. Also, people who live with mental illness tend to have fewer financial and social resources than those without, so perhaps insurers get away with it because patients don't have enough power to push back. The only people who benefit from the current mode of short-term inpatient care are insurance company stockholders. The priority is on saving money and not on patient care, often with deadly results.

After a full seven days in the hospital, I was discharged. I got to stay for a week because of the tireless advocacy of my parents, who cast aside their characteristic Midwest niceness in order to demand that the hospital keep me until I showed signs of improvement. I had never seen my mom yell at anyone the way she yelled at the social worker when, after three days, the hospital was ready for me to leave. I was in worse shape than when I was admitted, foggy from the half-dozen drugs in my system—one of which was lithium, which gave me a tremor and a charming tendency to drool. Six months earlier I had been backpacking around Europe, wearing a scarf in an attempt to look French, navigating train stations in Switzerland, trying to flirt in Italian. Now I slobbered and shook, could hardly stay awake, and sobbed all of my waking hours. I said over and over, "I'm not going to get better, I want to die." I wasn't well enough to go home.

Perhaps the most dangerous part of depression is this sureness that the sadness will never abate. The ability of the disease to push memories of happiness, even very recent happiness, to the outermost periphery of the mind, if not blacking it out entirely. Depression screamed in my face, "You will never feel any better! This is it, this is your life, in tatters. Just end it now." Depression, my worst enemy, assured me that I was an unbearable burden on my parents, my brother, my friends. That everyone would be so much happier if I just ended my life. That they only cared for me out of obligation.

How can anyone resist this logical-sounding voice, repeating over and over again, *You are worthless. You are hopeless. You will never recover. You are broken garbage, and everyone you love would be a million times better off if you no longer burdened the world with your existence.* This message on auto-replay, in synch with the breathtaking agony of sadness, the gut-wrenching sobs, the physical pain of despair. How does anyone survive depression? How did I?

First, it was deeply ingrained in my psyche that I was loved. One of my earliest memories is of walking out the back door, maybe six years old, and approaching my mom. She was sunbathing in a lounge chair, eyes closed, golden skin slick with baby oil, the most beautiful woman in the world. Prettier than Barbie and She-Ra combined. As I approached, she opened her eyes and her face creased with delight at my presence, cracking open with joy just because of me, just because I was there. I was probably there to bug her for a snack or tattle on my brother, but still—she was utterly thrilled to see me. Sliding her sun-warmed arms around me, imbuing me with her baby powder scent, I was loved completely just for existing. Not for being obedient (I wasn't) or possessing some amazing ability (nope), but just for being me.

My parents weren't perfect, but they were really good at unconditional love. And it wasn't just them—as the only granddaughter on my father's side, I had extended family marveling at my every move. Ballet recitals where I spun the wrong direction, forgot what I was doing, and stopped and picked my nose right up on stage were greeted with thunderous applause and an after-show ice cream sundae. My uncle scheduled his vacations around my choir concert schedule; my aunts spent months searching for a birthday present in the exact shade of pink I liked best. If I hadn't gotten depression, I might have turned out a spoiled monster. But having that thick, deep backlog of love made it hard for depression to convince me that I wasn't loved. There was just so much evidence to the contrary.

My second depression-fighting superpower was that I had seen people knocked down by this deep sadness before and survive. My dad would spend months depressed, and then one day I would come home from school and he would be fine. It happened again and again, every couple of years. It was confusing and anxiety provoking when he was sad, but seeing him recover was a powerful lesson. If he could do it, I could do it.

I also had faith. I was pretty mad at God, but wrestling with the Holy wasn't unusual for me. I didn't understand God's role in my life. As a child, I thought God decided everything—every leaf that fell from the tree was instructed to by God. When bad things like war happened, it was at God's command, and it was awful, but God worked in mysterious ways. I thought there was a reason that God made things like war happen and the reasons were just beyond my understanding. I thought that when I got older, I would understand.

Then, during my first year of college, my childhood friend Betsy died. Betsy and I grew up together, playing pranks during Sunday school classes, trying to sneak handfuls of cookies into our pockets at coffee hour. Betsy was whip-smart and hilarious, and just after Christmas break that year, she contracted meningitis and died. She was sick one day and gone the very next. It was an especially cruel death because two days before she died, she'd been home with her parents, both doctors, and if she'd had any symptoms then they would have gotten her to the hospital in plenty of time.

Betsy's death sent me into a spiral of doubt about God. There couldn't be an upside to Betsy's death. She was a warm, kind person who, despite our shared love of practical jokes, never hurt anyone. I couldn't keep believing that God had a plan when the plan seemed full of mess-ups like Betsy's death. I wanted answers, not mystery. For the first time, I didn't trust God.

In the weeks after Betsy's death, I wandered my college campus feeling numb with a sharp edge of pain. I only wanted to be outside, outside being where I usually found God, but it was a bitterly cold winter. Thick snow covered every inch of the campus. My fellow undergrads sledded down the slick hills on stolen cafeteria trays, whooping with delight, but I heard only my feet crunching in the snow. As my toes began to tingle with frostbite, I made my way into the basement of the campus chapel, where there was always hot tea and sometimes even cookies. As I stirred honey into my tea, the college minister came out of his office to say hi.

Reverend Jerry had an open face and extremely thick, long, gray eyebrows that made me think of a Muppet. He was pretty radical for our college and for a Presbyterian. He joked that tenure made him theologically bold. I admired him for being pro-gay and pro-choice in rural Ohio, where those positions made him unpopular. I hadn't ever spoken to him one on one, but when he saw my red eyes, he raised his bushy eyebrows in concern, and my whole Betsy story came out.

Jerry quickly gathered that I was grieving not just the loss of a friend I had known nearly my whole life but the loss of my life's theology as well. I believed God had a reason for everything she did, that there was a plan for everyone and everything, and that God loved me more than I could imagine. But if God loved me so much, why was Betsy gone? And didn't God love Betsy? What good could come of her death? Was this whole God thing just a story, like Santa Claus and the Easter Bunny?

Jerry said, "Maybe." What kind of a minister says "maybe" when you ask if God is real? He reminded me that the Bible was an anthology of ideas people had about God. Some of it was probably true, some false, most of it somewhere between the two. But, Jerry explained, for him God wasn't a puppetmaster. God didn't create a script and then force us to all act out our parts. We have free will. God was sad about Betsy's death too, Jerry believed, but God wept with me in my grief.

I liked the idea of free will when it came to Betsy's death. Free will meant that God herself hadn't decided that my kind, funny friend would die. God didn't script out how all of human history would go and then use us as puppets to act it out. Maybe, I thought, God had set the universe in motion and then let every creature make its own choices. Maybe God whispered in our ear: "Remember to be kind!" and hoped for the best. This was a gigantic shift in how I thought about God, and it allowed my faith to grow in new directions. It was a big comfort to think of God as beside me in my grief, not causing it.

But a few years later, depressed and anxious, I wondered: if God wasn't making all the decisions, what was the point of prayer? Since my first panic attack, I'd been praying fervently. I wanted a way out of this painful condition, whether by pharmaceuticals or the supernatural. If God was a kindly Creator weeping with me, did it matter if I prayed? I was mad at my new version of God for not being all-powerful. I wanted a God who could throw her weight around. I wanted God to declare from the heavens that I would suffer no more and send down lightning bolts to decimate my mental illness. I wanted the God of the Hebrew Bible parting the waters for me, not a friend to cry with.

Still, I had faith. I believed in God. I felt her dancing in the tree limbs on windy days, in the crystalline snow, in the tenacity of the first purple crocus every spring. She was in my parents, in how well they loved me, in my brother quietly comforting me during visiting hours. Even if God didn't make any sense, she was still with me.

Finally, there was my faith community. At age two, I began attending the First Baptist Church of Dayton, a liberal American Baptist church in the city center. From toddlerhood, I was tightly woven into a community of people who not only loved me unconditionally but also held me accountable. I knew every member of the church, and they were with me for all my struggles. They were there when I almost failed algebra (Mr. Wingam offered to tutor me before Sunday worship every week, and I managed to get a C). They were with me when my dad got angry at coffee hour and started screaming about who-knows-what. That day and in the weeks to follow, people violated the mind-your-own-business rule that plagues so many churches and asked me if he yelled at home, if he hit me, if he was abusive. In ways both subtle and not, adults young and old let me know that it wasn't okay for anyone to mistreat me and that they were a safe person for me to talk to.

On Youth Sunday the year before, I had given a sermon on the holy power of Mary: Mary as a gatekeeper for God, Mary as Goddess. It was radical stuff, even in my very liberal congregation—we were still Baptists, after all. But the congregation listened politely and followed up at coffee hour with questions I hadn't considered. They were open to what would have been heresy in similar congregations. They loved me even if I had wild ideas.

When I faced peer pressure, I remembered that I had my church youth group friends, and so it didn't matter if these school people rejected me. When a guy at school asked me to a dance and I said no, he started following me home, driving by our house at odd hours, leaving me disturbing notes. Ashamed and afraid that I had somehow inadvertently led him on, I called my minister Jacque. She told me right away that it wasn't my fault and that I deserved to be safe. She helped me figure out how to talk to my parents, who then talked to the school principal. The guy backed off. I loved my church family, but I also owed them—they would be devastated if I ended my life. They would wonder what they could have done. They would miss me. Even if I spent the rest of my life in a depressed haze, I needed to spare them my death. They loved me so well. I needed to survive and love them back.

It was at church that I first started to believe I might get well. I was discharged from the hospital on a Saturday and dragged to church by my parents the day after. My name was on the "please pray for . . ." list in the newsletter so everyone knew what was up with me. I didn't want to face them. I was afraid that they would reject me, think I had failed somehow. What if they thought God was punishing me or that they would be tainted if they were near me? My fears were the depression talking, that feeling of worthlessness that comes with the disease. I didn't feel like I deserved love from these people who had helped me countless times before. So in my mind, I set this church service up as a test: if these people, my church family, pushed me away, I would know I really was broken.

I walked into a love fest. No one yelled "sinner" at me or tried to cast out Satan. Lots of people hugged me, told me how much they loved me, said they were there for me. My former babysitter, whom I idolized, gave me a journal with a long letter that detailed her experience with depression and hoped writing would help me (it did and does). A youth group friend gave me a potted daffodil, brave yellow hope in the winter grayscape. Everyone seemed genuinely glad to see me. They said they were praying for me and told me to call anytime, even if it was 4 AM. I could feel their love like warm sun thawing the snow. I would make it through this.

My trudge through depression was far from over, but knowing I was loveable, that even when broken, I belonged, made me resist committing suicide. Even when every moment was physical and emotional agony, I held onto the memory of that daffodil blooming in the wintertime.

10.

Off the Roof

I WOULDN'T HAVE BLAMED Drew for bailing out. One spring evening, after I was released from the hospital but still not really stabilized, Drew and I sat on the porch roof of my off-campus house. I had just returned to school triumphant, ready to get back to normal life. But the panic attacks were ruthless in cutting through my medications. The medication side effects were making me feel wretched. It was less a triumphant return than a big mistake.

I was crying; Drew was whispering soothing things. I didn't feel like I could take the pain inside my body anymore. I was choking on it, on the sadness that had been welling up all day. The grief started out as it always did, awful but manageable. But it grew and grew. It was a searing-hot ball with jagged edges, moving from my stomach into my throat. I couldn't breathe. I gagged on nothing. The pain had to be expelled.

I glanced off the roof and saw a gently sloping bank of green grass, radiant in the late-afternoon sunlight. I wanted to jump off the roof and onto the grass. I was sure that I would survive, but maybe break my legs, and in that physical pain my emotional pain would be released. The broken-leg pain would make sense, unlike the jagged ball inside me. Jumping seemed like the sanest option. I didn't want to die. I wanted my pain to have an outlet.

Drew saw me narrow my eyes, a sure sign that I was plotting. He saw me looking at the ground and grabbed me around the waist, pulling me horizontal on the roof, immobilized. He rapidly reasoned with me: "You know this isn't what God wants. God wants you to live. Come on, Kate, don't do this to me. I love you so much. Don't, Babe, don't. Please don't." He was crying and I realized I was too. We climbed back inside the window and went downstairs—I didn't want to be high enough to jump off anything if the urge arose again.

Downstairs, my housemates, my very best friends, were watching a movie. We all tearfully decided that I should go back to the hospital in Zanesville, an hour or so away. The whole gang tagged along. My parents met us there. I kept repeating, again and again, "I don't want to die, I just want the pain gone." Drew understood, but the nurses were wary. They wanted to put me in a straightjacket, like in a horror movie. They wanted to put me in a padded room in this crazy jacket with my arms bound.

"Don't you think you'd be more comfortable?" one nurse cooed soothingly.

"No. I am not that person. I am not a crazy person," I replied.

"Well, sane people don't try to jump off roofs," she snapped back.

We stared at each other, both sure that the other person was off her rocker. Finally, the doctor entered, said a sedative would be more effective than all that tying up, and the nurse huffed out.

Before I got my sedative and headed to my room, my housemates came in to talk with me. I was weepy and snot-covered, weak with fatigue. Lynn, who always took charge, said that everyone loved me and was worried about me. That was nice to hear, but she continued by saying that since it was our senior year and everyone was just trying to graduate and move on, it would be best if I didn't come back to our house. That they were trying to enjoy senior year and I was too stressful to be around.

I was speechless. These women had become my best friends. We had shared the most intimate details of our lives in late-night conversations, confessed our deepest fears. And now one of mine was coming true—I was being dumped by people I loved. I was too broken to share their home.

The mean nurse bustled back in with my sedative and hustled them out. I went to my room and slept deeply. But for years afterward, I struggled with that conversation, that friendship termination. I felt disposable. I had been lucky with friendships in my life up to that point, and for the first time wondered if any of those friends had really loved me. Would anyone want to be friends with me now that I was crazy?

11.

Electric Hallelujah

I WOKE UP to my roommate's soft crying, a gentle, pleading sound. "Help, help," she murmured over and over, her seated posture slumped, eyes full of tears. She looked at me questioningly as I sat up in bed. "Where am I?" she asked.

For three days we had shared a room in the psych ward. She was forty-one, short and plump, with huge brown eyes. She had a husband, a handsome, stocky guy who always looked worried, and two small boys with her big eyes. They came to visit every evening during visitation hours and cried the entire time, which wasn't unusual. People aren't super cheery in the psych ward.

I was just waking up, but already my roommate had gone through her first electroshock treatment. I slept through their taking her away, but my doctor had warned me that she would wake up confused. Electroshock treatment was just beginning to be discussed as an option for me. It had been a worst-case scenario just a few months before: an unlikely need, a last-ditch effort in case nothing else worked. But by April nothing else had worked, for me or my roommate, and so while I was sleeping through the morning sunrise, she was being zapped with electricity.

My doctor described it as turning off a computer and turning it back on, the classic tech support response when an operating system is malfunctioning. Of course, in 2001, desktop computers took a few minutes to shut down and then another few to reboot. Meanwhile, there was a low whirling sound and a light gray screen. That's all I could imagine when I thought of electroshock—that gray screen and low whine. What if I get stuck there? Is the gray screen death? "Just brain death," my doctor tried to assure me. "Your brain dies for a second, and then we restart it." Just brain death? That was not reassuring.

"There is no way you are doing that to me," I replied, and she just raised her eyebrows as if to say, *We will see.*

My roommate didn't know where she was, so I reminded her: "Zanesville Psych Ward," immediately wishing that I had used the more polite term, behavioral health unit. She didn't seem to register my answer and began picking tiny bits of cotton off of her pink calico hospital gown.

"Who am I?" she asked anxiously. Shit. I didn't think she was that messed up. I wondered if I should call for a nurse. I put my feet on the icy floor and started for the door, but her eyes went wide: "Nonono! Don't leave me!"

Time for compulsive prayer. "Dear God please get me out of this shithole I hate this what the fuck—okay I need you down here tell me what to say Amen." My roommate was still looking at me, so I sat on her bed, took her cold hand, and said her name. Told her that she had been here a few days, that every day her husband and kids visited. She looked shocked—no recognition of having a family. "Dear Jesus," I prayed, "what level of Hell is this? Could you get on this, please? Was this part of your divine plan?" My anger at God skyrocketed.

I told her that she had a family who came every day and that they loved her so much—adored her, really. That her sons looked just like her, that they were sweet boys. That her husband was handsome, which made her laugh. That she lived nearby, that she was having a rough spell—that's what everyone says to psych patients, it's a "rough spell"— and that soon she would be back to normal.

"They love me?" was her only reply. "They love you," I repeated, because when you are confused and sick, what else is there? Some people loved her. Hallelujah. She didn't remember them, but they loved her. "They love you, I promise. So much."

"Okay," she said doubtfully, and lay down, closing her eyes, immediately sleeping. I gently released her hand and slid into my own bed, sobbing into the pillow. Where was God in all of this hell? Were we forgotten? Forsaken? *For God so loved the world that he created people with broken minds, so that they could suffer without end and break their family's hearts. Amen.*

All of the old religious traditions told stories. These stories were not understood to be fact, but a parable, a tale taught to teach a moral lesson. Stories were told because few people could read, and even fewer could write, but everyone enjoyed a good tale told in front of the campfire. And so children learned the stories of their religious heritage from adults and passed them on for generations.

The story of Jacob and Esau is especially juicy, like reality television from 1400 BCE. Rebekah, the twin's mother, felt them fighting in her womb, and while Esau was born first, Jacob came out holding Esau's heel. Being born first meant that Esau inherited the family herds, tents, and servants, which made Jacob furious. Also infuriating was that while mom Rebekah preferred Jacob, dad Isaac preferred Esau. As a teenager, Esau comes in from herding exhausted, sweaty, and sore. He asks his brother to get him a bowl of red lentil stew, and Jacob says, "Sure, if I can have your birthright. Sure, if I can inherit everything from Dad, taking on the rights of the oldest brother." And Esau, who is impulsive and rather foolish, says "Sure—take all of it, just give me those lentils." I can hear the people around the campfire going, "What?! Come on, Esau, don't do it!" I can see moms leaning over to whisper to dads, "See, this is why we have to treat the kids equally. This is why we have to make as big a deal out of Raina's soccer game as Max's science fair, even if we think soccer is boring."

But Esau, immature and unappreciative of his parents, who are a big deal in these stories, turns over his birthright for soup. Of course, later he is furious with Jacob, so furious that Jacob flees for his life. Rebekah sets Jacob up with a job with her cousin Laban, far away, and he is gone for twenty-something years. This hasn't turned out the way Jacob had hoped—he is a servant in Laban's camp. After twenty or so years, though, Jacob is in possession of considerable wealth. Isaac calls his son home, and Jacob sends word to Esau, along with a mountain of gifts, hoping that Esau won't kill him.

Esau says he will meet with Jacob. Lest this all seem pretty peacenik, both brothers prepare as if they are going into battle, just in case. Jacob even has his family approach from two directions so that if one group is attacked by Esau's troops, the other group will survive to carry on the family line. Not a lot of trust between these brothers.

Jacob and his extended family walk for many weeks to get to Jacob's homeland. On the last night of the journey the family crosses a river, but Jacob stays behind to camp alone and think on this final night before he reunites with his brother Esau. And here by the river, in the middle of nowhere, a creature appears, maybe an angel, and tackles Jacob. They wrestle all night. They are a well-matched pair, both equally strong and skilled, and though they both use all of their abilities, neither can seem to win.

So day is breaking, and a common motif in these stories is that angels, or God, or any supernatural being, can only be out at night. So the angel whacks Jacob really hard in the thigh, permanently injuring him, trying to end the fight. But Jacob still doesn't give up, and the angel says, "Let go of me, the sun is starting to rise." Jacob says, "No, I won't, unless you bless me."

Now, around the campfire, this must have caused quite a stir. This is the Hebrew Bible, after all, where God is as likely to smite your whole tribe as to bless you. This isn't a God you want to mess with. What is Jacob thinking? Is he brave or just really stupid?

The angel says, "Who are you?" And Jacob gives him his name. The angel says, "From now on you will be known as Israel, which means wrestles with God, because you are one stubborn human!" Jacob then has the gall to ask, "Who are you?"

The angel responds with, "Who do you think you are that you get to ask me questions?" and disappears. The only evidence of this wrestling is Jacob's aching thigh, which makes him limp for the rest of his life.

Israel. One who wrestles with the mystery of God.

Jacob continues on to meet Esau, scared to pieces that he is about to be murdered by his brother. But when Esau sees Jacob, he embraces him, tears streaming down his face.

As if this wasn't enough of a surprise for our fireside audience, Jacob then sees the face of God in Esau.

A footnote: until this moment in the Jewish story, God was called Adonai, which meant absolute ruler, boss over all the other bosses. Adonai is plural to connote that this isn't just the king, but the king of kings. This is probably the version of God we think of when we think of the God who sends famines and floods in the Old Testament, or Hebrew Bible.

But in Esau, Jacob sees Elohim, a much different vision of the divine. This is the holiness that is in every person. This is brand new to the folks listening to this story in 1450 BCE: God within us, not just ruling over us. Huge news— a radical shift from God out there to God within us. God above us to God right in here. Let's let that sink in.

God, the angry grandfather in the sky, making all the rules, was Adonai. But Jacob sees Elohim, a different holiness. The divine within every person and every living creature. The divine in his brother, who he has hated since birth. Elohim is genderless, formless, and timeless. The god energy that connects. The god energy that is love. For Jacob, it is unlikely that Elohim, god within us, replaced Adonai, but rather became an equal way of understanding the divine. Jacob probably believed that God was both outside of us and inside of us.

For Martin Buber, Adonai didn't exist at all. Martin Buber was a Jewish Humanist philosopher who called

Jacob's experience with Esau the "I-Thou encounter." Buber, born in Austria in 1878, was nominated for the Nobel Prize in Literature ten times and the Nobel Peace Prize seven times for his work on a state of Israel with an equal Palestinian state. Buber said that the only way humans could encounter divinity, or universality or infinity, was through the I-thou encounter: the moment when we connect with another person or animal and realize that they are as significant as we are, as real as we are. When we meet as equals but don't want anything from each other, we can sense this infinity that some people call God.

For Buber, this infinity was God, all of God. No Adonai. He didn't believe in a King of Kings or a divine ruler but in a universal, unending love that connects living things when we can put down all the weight of our egoist needs and our desires from other people. Elohim. The holy mystery within us.

Buber believed this holy I-thou experience could happen to anyone. He said divinity can be glimpsed between two lovers, between an observer and a cat, between himself and a tree, between two strangers on a train. The I-thou moment isn't just for monks on a mountain or romantic love—it can happen any time we connect with another being without seeking anything from them. As soon as our ego takes back over, that glimpse of holiness is gone, but we can experience the divine again when we are ready to let our guard down.

When Jacob wrestled with the angel, he wrestled with his ideas about God: his holy inheritance, the God his father worshipped. The God that was outside of humanity, ruling over us from without. He wrestled with those ideas about God and came up with his own theology: God inside of us. He wouldn't let go of his theological struggle until he had a new understanding. And so he witnessed God not far away in a holy realm but right in the face of his brother. His brother who did dumb things, like trade his birthright for lentil stew. His brother who forgave him. There was holiness in this imperfect creature.

A FEW HOURS LATER, my hospital roommate woke up clearheaded. I didn't tell her that we had talked earlier and she didn't seem to remember. She was hopeful that the electroshock had worked and giddy that it was over, that she had made it through the procedure. She was excited to see her family. She praised Jesus and thanked me for praying for her. I accepted her thanks without telling her how much cursing my prayers had involved, more demands made of an absent God than polite requests and praise. Despite her outward piety, I imagined her prayers were similar.

A few days later, she went home, her boys bickering over who got to carry her duffle bag, her husband with his arm protectively around her shoulders. She was happy; the electroshock seemed to have worked. For all of two days, she hadn't had a hysterical bout of crying, so the insurance company decided it was time to get her out of there. I never saw her again, as is often the case in the psych ward—patients get so close but only know each other by first name and then are gone. I still prayed for her, prayed to the God I was furious with, because she had asked me to. Because love is stronger than death, even stronger than memory.

> Set me as a seal upon your heart,
>   as a seal upon your arm;
>   for love is stronger than death,
>   passion fiercer than the grave.
>   Its flashes are flashes of fire,
>   a raging flame.
> Many waters cannot quench love,
>   neither can floods drown it.
>   If one offered for love
>   all the wealth of one's house,
>   it would be utterly scorned.

That day in the hospital was not the first or last time I would wrestle with God. It can be so hard to understand why people have to suffer. Why would God make faulty brains that sometimes get stuck in sad mode? Sometimes I am too angry with Adonai to keep that line of communication open. If I could physically wrestle an incarnation of Adonai, I would be up for it, just to get out some anger and frustration. But Elohim and I are always on good terms. It is so much easier to see God in the eyes of my fellow humans. It was in my roommate, even when she didn't remember her own name. Holiness was plentiful in her children and her husband; God practically burst out of them. I might wrestle Adonai, but I embrace Elohim.

12.

Sharon Jumped

SHARON JUMPED OFF the roof of the parking garage. I feel like I should put a trigger warning before that statement, but by that logic, this whole damn book needs a trigger warning. Sharon jumped off the parking garage during lunch break after I avoided her because I didn't want to go to lunch with her. She jumped off the fifth floor and smashed all her bones and died what is reportedly an excruciating death.

We were outpatient therapy buddies, released from the psych ward for good behavior, but not well enough to be left alone during the day, when whoever was responsible for us was at work. My parents had used all their vacation days and sick days trying to keep me alive, so now the hospital babysat me by day and they took over at five. Sharon was in her thirties and had a husband and kids, so at five she

114

went back to pretending to be sane until the kids went to bed, at which time she cried herself to sleep beside her sympathetic husband.

The outpatient crowd was different from the psych ward: fewer poor people, no homeless people. Outpatient day camp required fairly good insurance. We were a group of middle-class people on a psychic break from the reality of suburban homes and office jobs. I don't know how Sharon and I ended up eating lunch together—perhaps it was our utter fury at being depressed. Many depressed people are too sad to get angry, but Sharon and I raged against our illness, the doctors and the therapists trying to help us, and the side effects of our pharmaceutical cocktails. We were pissed off at anything we could think of to be pissed off about. That kind of rage bonds people. Plus, we both swore a lot.

If you are getting the impression that I was some kind of psych patient bad boy, I was not. I was still hyper-religious and a people pleaser. But three hospitalizations had worn out 80 percent of my optimism and 90 percent of my goodwill toward medical professionals. I heard "This med always works, don't worry, you'll be back to normal in two weeks" dozens of times, and it was never true. Whatever magic trick fixed other people's brains didn't work on mine. I couldn't help but roll my eyes. I was my good-Ohio-girl version of a bad boy, which meant I swore generally but not at people, and I looked skeptical instead of enthusiastic.

Sharon had me beat in the skepticism department. She had only been hospitalized twice—lightweight—but she was pretty sure she wasn't ever getting better. This is where having a depressed dad has its advantages: he had been depressed, got better, got depressed, got better, etc., forever. I figured I would get better. Maybe not for long, but for a while. Then I would get depressed and get better again. It wasn't ideal, but it sure beat Sharon's faith that while her life had been pretty okay pre-depression—she felt lucky to have her husband and kids—now that party was over. She believed that while this felt like hell, it would probably get worse.

My dad's cycle of depression and recovery is probably why Sharon ate lunch with me most days. She liked to hear about him getting better. But one Tuesday she cried hysterically the whole time we were eating. She talked about all the specific ways she could end her life. She had worked out all the details. And so when she was in the restroom, I went to the outpatient office and told on her. I reported that Sharon seemed suicidal and maybe should be locked back in the hospital. The therapist thanked me for being a tattletale and said they would look into it. And he reminded me of something I kept hearing: that we had to each prioritize our own healing. That in group therapy situations like this it was easier to worry about each other than to do our own hard work of recovering. So, the therapist said, it's nice you care about Sharon, but quit avoiding dealing with your shit by worrying about someone else's shit.

That night I asked my dad if he could meet me for lunch the next day. He worked nearby and always bought me cinnamon candy in the hospital cafeteria. Plus, it gave me an excuse to not eat with Sharon. Hearing about the many ways she had imagined offing herself set my suicidal ideation on fire—I couldn't think of anything but self-harm. I was following instructions and working on my own shit.

The next day, Sharon was hysterical for much of the morning session. I felt sorry for her but also wondered where she got the energy to stay in anxiety attack level 10 for so long. My worst anxiety attacks were an hour or so—after that, I was too exhausted to feel anything and just became numb. But all morning, she wailed and shook. It was awful. Maybe she was suffering a lot more than I was. It's hard to rank misery. Plus, I can't speak for all depressed people, but mine made me pretty self-centered—I thought I was the most depressed person ever in the history of depression. But maybe that's just me.

When lunchtime arrived, I shot her a sympathetic smile and then broke eye contact. I rushed off to meet my dad even as I saw she was moving toward me. I wouldn't have ignored her if I'd known what she was going to do next. But I snuck off for a pleasant lunch with my dad, some cinnamon candy, and his corny jokes. And when I got back to the therapy room, everyone but Sharon was there. I assumed that she was back in the hospital, back in the locked psych ward, and I felt relieved for her. Not that psych was fun, but it was safe. I wanted her to be safe.

The afternoon session continued as normal, with the exception of the therapist getting called out of the room a lot by other medical staff. That night my heart, that traitor, felt a little lighter. I felt a bit more hopeful. That night I told my parents that I felt like I wouldn't need another week in outpatient group. I felt like I could stay home by myself. I wasn't going to want to die. My parents were uncharacteristically nonplussed about my announcement and just said we would wait and see.

The outpatient psych office had called them that afternoon. They knew about Sharon. It must have been brutal, not telling me. But the therapist wanted to tell us all together, in our safe little classroom. So the next morning when I arrived in group, there were way more therapists than normal. There were boxes of tissues everywhere. I want to claim that at that moment I knew Sharon was dead, but I didn't. I was thinking about me. So when our therapist finally said that he had a very sad announcement, that unfortunately Sharon had ended her life, a wave of gray covered my vision. I heard a loud ringing, like an elementary school fire alarm, that erased every other noise. My fingers and toes tingled. I fainted for a minute or two, then gasped for air, like a drowning woman breaking the surface of the water.

Excruciating pain. Utter hopelessness. Fury. But I was speechless, not a word getting through the cement block stuck in my throat. Just gasps as I struggled for air.

I don't remember the rest of the afternoon. The next morning, we had a memorial service, just our group, in the hospital chapel. A group of nuns led it. One held my hand and said that Sharon was lucky to have me as a friend. So lucky, I thought, to have a friend that avoided her as she daydreamed about her own demise. What a super friend I was, eating cinnamon candy and rolling my eyes at Dad's jokes while she took the elevator to the fifth floor of the parking garage. What was I doing when she looked over the edge? When she climbed over the cement guardrail? When her body came to a full stop?

Elohim was dead. I saw God in Sharon, a smart-assed, sarcastic God. A tell-it-like-it-is, no-bullshit God. My faith smashed into the pavement, and I walked away in a wave of gray. Sharon's kids had no mother. How did her husband tell them? What kind of a God was this?

At the memorial service, a nun read the 23rd Psalm:

The Lord is my Shepherd; I shall not want.
He maketh me to lie down in green pastures:
He leadeth me beside the still waters.
He restoreth my soul:
He leadeth me in the paths of righteousness for
    His name' sake.

Yea, though I walk through the valley of the
shadow of death,
I will fear no evil: For thou art with me;
Thy rod and thy staff, they comfort me.
Thou preparest a table before me in the presence
of mine enemies;
Thou annointest my head with oil; My cup
runneth over.

Surely goodness and mercy shall follow me all
the days of my life,
and I will dwell in the House of the Lord
forever.

Fuck you, I thought, talking to God in my head. "Fuck you," I said out loud, talking to the nun in the chapel. "Worst Shepherd ever. Where were Sharon's green pastures? Wasn't her head good enough to anoint with oil? What about her fucking kids? You going to shepherd them too, God? You know, since their mom is dead?" The nun just looked at me sadly. When you are super depressed and your therapy buddy commits suicide, people cut you a lot of breaks. You can say nearly anything. I walked out of the chapel, throwing up in the bushes outside. That was the end of me and God for a while.

This probably feels like a pretty fast spiritual shift, from my incredible gratitude to God for healing my roommate after electroshock to my fierce anger at God for Sharon's violent death. It was quick. I was twenty-one and in deep despair. In a time of crisis, my devotion to God became conditional. I didn't want theological mystery and holy curiosity; I wanted the big guy in the sky to protect me and my friends from scary, deadly shit like depression and suicide. I was a good kid, I was nice to the weirdos at school, I didn't lie or cheat or steal. I did unto others as I would want them to do to me. I prayed, I read my Bible, I didn't have sex. I wanted a payoff for my good behavior.

JAMES FOWLER was a United Methodist minister, a professor of theology and human development at Emory University, and, from what I hear, a really nice guy. He developed this idea of "stages of faith," levels of spiritual formation that fit with Jean Piaget's stages of cognitive development. Fowler's theory is that as we age, we go through fairly predictable phases in thinking about religion and faith. From birth to around age two, we are in the Primal or Undifferentiated stage. We experience either safety and love, and therefore feel that the universe is a safe and loving place, or neglect and abuse, and think that the universe is terrible. Then, from around age three to seven (the Intuitive-Projective stage), it's hard for kids to see the difference between magic, religion, and reality. So, if they hear a story about God flooding the Earth and killing everyone but Noah and the inhabitants of the ark, they think that God is a villain and might get really freaked out every time it rains. Then they might ask if Noah can come over for dinner so they can ask for a place on the ark and then want to invite Santa too. Kids in this stage are drawn to epic tales, but fairytales, their dreams, and reality are all a hazy mix. In many ways, small children are like people on psychedelics.

Next is Mythic-Literal faith, which I see in the elementary school–aged kids at church. They are all about fairness: good things happen to good people, bad guys get punished. Deities are anthropomorphized—they look and act like people. This is why I get so many questions about the Buddha getting cold because he is usually pictured without a shirt. This is why my niece thinks God is a man (well, that and the damn patriarchy).

Then comes the stage most people stay in: Synthetic-Conventional faith. It starts in adolescence and is based on conformity. Usually it involves people hunkering down with the faith they grew up in. They identify with the group's identity and don't let any doubts in; they might get angry or defensive if their beliefs are questioned. My favorite part about this stage is that people don't have to hunker down with religion specifically—they can have loyal, unquestioning faith in a sports team or a frat. Next time you see people getting in a fight over college football, tell them to quit being so Synthetic-Conventional. Then duck.

I was really good at the Synthetic-Conventional stage of faith. I was Christian, as were 99 percent of the people I knew, and I got a lot of positive feedback for going to church. My teachers were happy to hear about my faith at my public school, where nearly everyone was also Christian. When weird inconsistencies came up, like our church welcoming gay people and my friend's church, also Christian, condemning gay people, I squashed those uncomfortable thoughts down as hard as possible. When people asked why God would create Jesus to atone for humanity's sins when God could just forgive those sins without all the gory crucifixion stuff, and why God would create people who were imperfect and then be so angry that they were imperfect, my heart raced and I refused to engage. My loyalty was with Christianity. I was team Jesus, but I wasn't able to consider conflicting ideas within my faith or handle critical comments about my theology.

I wasn't looking to change my ideas about God. But then Betsy died, and I was shoved right into the next stage: Individuative-Reflective, the least fun phase. It was an angsty, painful place, where all my unquestioning faith was blown up by doubts. Was faith bullshit? I felt like a trick had been played on me, and I was embarrassed by my previous public devotion to Christianity. Surely, I thought, anyone with a brain could see the contradictions in the Bible. How had I missed them? Not to mention the differences between how

Jesus said to live and how Christians actually live today. I felt foolish. I had walked around proudly proclaiming my Christianity while not noticing the shallowness of my own understanding. People must have been laughing behind my back. I was a chump.

Plus, I didn't fit in with the group I loved fitting in with. I liked my Christian friends. I liked our corny church camp songs, our campfire testimonials, our lack of jadedness. We were innocent and optimistic. But now all of that seemed childish. I didn't want to stand in a big circle and sing "Here I Am, Lord" while exchanging meaningful looks with my fellow college students who were passing around a loaf of communion bread. The bread was from the grocery down the street, and the song was meaningless in my new world where God could let illness steal your friend's life. Did my Christian friends, standing with me in that communion circle, understand how worthless faith had been when Betsy was dying?

Lots of people are pushed into the Individuative-Reflective phase by moving away from home, traveling abroad, or taking a philosophy class in college. When we are outside of the bubble of our ideologically alike community, we start to see how fragile our beliefs are in a complex, adult world. My naïve Synthetic-Conventional faith would have perished even if Betsy had lived. It was an inevitable transition. After Betsy's death, my college minister helped me to see that I could stay a Christian and question theology, practice, and even religious leaders. He introduced me to other doubters who were coping with the same losses as I was. The maturation of my spirituality was painful, but I was staying in the fight. I wasn't giving up on God just yet. Just on unquestioning faith.

But a few years later, the trauma of losing my own emotional health was enough to make me an angry atheist. Somewhere after the three hospitalizations and billionth crying jag, the suicidal ideation and the antidepressants that worked on everyone except me, I was just pissed off. All my life I had talked to God (in the praying way, not in the delusional way) and felt a calm, loving presence envelop me. But in the past few months, I felt only loneliness. Had despair come between me and God, or was God just a part of my imagination? I felt furious with a God I claimed I didn't believe in. I felt abandoned by a fairytale I was embarrassed that I had ever needed. "You stupid fool, you batshit idiot," I said to myself over and over. "Even if God existed, God certainly doesn't love you. Look at your garbage-fire life. No one loves you, including your imaginary deity."

Sharon was dead. I was just barely alive, but my spirituality was extinguished. Life was a meaningless trudge toward the obliteration of death, as I told anyone who asked. (I was super fun to be around.) My mind was obsessed with suicide. Violent thoughts ran on a loop through every minute of my waking life. But seeing the impact that Sharon's death had on our therapy group made me feel tremendously guilty at even thinking about suicide. Now I know that suicidal ideation (obsessive, repetitive suicidal thoughts) isn't necessarily a sign of suicidality but more of anxiety and obsessive thinking. Back then, when I wasn't anxious about my violent mind, I berated myself that I could be so selfish as to even think about suicide. How could I do that to the people who cared about me? Shockingly, guilt did not help my recovery.

13.

No Resurrection for Cool Girls

I DIDN'T BELIEVE IN GOD, but I was obsessed with resurrection. I wanted a full restoration of my body and soul. I wanted to push aside the stone and exit the shadowy tomb of death. I longed to be the woman I was before the Big Depression began. But I'm not Jesus, and my recovery was less an Easter Sunday miracle and more a slow trudge to the new normal. I felt awful, then slightly less awful, every day. It took years to feel mostly okay, most of the time.

I was twenty-two years old and was about six weeks out of the hospital. Sharon was four weeks dead. The pharmaceutical cocktail had begun to work on my brain, and I went from craving the oblivion of death to thinking that maybe— not certainly, but maybe—this living business wasn't a completely rotten deal. It happened in teeny increments. One day I was in the car, my dad driving me home from out-patient therapy appointment number 1,000, and I heard a new song that I liked, and I smiled. It was such an odd feeling, my muscles unused to turning my mouth upward. Next, I was reading a novel and I laughed out loud—a real laugh, loud enough to pleasantly surprise my parents. Then food started to taste good again. As my body adjusted to the medication side effects and the depression eased, a few bits of all that I'd lost began to return.

Still, I longed for the joy at just existing that used to bub-ble inside of me. I remembered happiness but found it elu-sive. I was so tired. Tired emotionally, from the intense inner work of psychotherapy and learning new ways to manage my chronic anxiety. A huge amount of energy was expended to combat my suicidal ideation. The seemingly unending cycle of disturbing visions of myself dead after some horrif-ically violent, self-inflicted act tormented my waking hours. Despite the break in the relentless sorrow of depression, I was still plagued by unstable moods and dark thoughts.

This isn't an unusual predicament for survivors of a cri-sis. I was through the worst of the depression. Still, I was traumatized by my own recent history and feared that any second the huge waves of sadness would return. Having crawled onto shore, I feared that I was too tired, should I get sucked into the undertow again, to make it back out.

Bedraggled and bruised, I tried to imagine what life would look like, what adulthood would look like, now that I was saddled with these psychiatric curses and living with my parents, perhaps indefinitely. And I was physically tired. After months of hardly moving, I finally listened when my therapist suggested that exercise could slow my panic attacks. I began walking, then running. It seemed the worst of the anxiety couldn't keep up—I felt a panic attack coming and grabbed my shoes. Running down the sidewalk, my heart had a reason to race, and the feelings of terror stayed in the periphery rather than taking over.

Still, I craved the resurrection of my body and spirit. In my mind, the Easter story was about Jesus as resilient to death. Sure, some awful people had tortured and murdered him. And most of his friends had abandoned him, fleeing the second their own lives were imperiled. But three days after his broken corpse was deposited in a cave tomb, he emerged unscathed. I pictured Jesus waking up refreshed, as if from a long nap, shaking out his limbs, brushing off his clothes, and pushing away the stone that separated him from the living. Strolling out into the morning sunshine, ready to begin ministry again.

Ten years later, in seminary, I learned that it wasn't that simple. The Christian Bible has radically different versions of what the resurrection of Jesus really meant. Did Jesus walk the earth in the same body as before his death? Did only his soul live on? Was he resurrected in the sense that his inspiration lingered in the hearts of his followers, inspiring them to continue to spread his theology? We know that

Jesus was Jewish and that most Jews at that time believed in the resurrection of the soul but not the body. Some Jews believed that immediately after death, a person's soul went to either a place of punishment or a place of reward, depending on the virtue of their earthly deeds. Other Jews believed that the souls of the dead would rise when the Kingdom of God arrived, in the end times. A few believed in bodily resurrection, but it was a rare idea.

The resurrection debate intensified as Christianity spread into cultures more attuned to Greek and Roman thought. Among theologians who believed in Jesus' bodily resurrection—because a spirit needs a body, none of this ghost business—the debate was over why Jesus would be stuck with his earthly body. After all, having been tortured and then crucified, his body wasn't in great shape. And even before all of that, he was in his thirties, which was pretty old back then, and so his body would have all the aches and pains we associate with old age. They argued that it would be better for him to get a perfect new body to fit with his resurrected soul. But where would the body come from? And could this body be made of the regular old stuff that human bodies are made from? Some theologians believed that Jesus' new body must be made a of substance holier than anything human but not quite as holy as the stuff making up God's body. If God had a body.

Every question begat a new series of questions. If Jesus was impervious to death, then why the three-day wait period for resurrection? Was that Jesus' choice? Or God's choice? Where was Jesus' soul during those three days? Was he really dead or just under a spell to make him seem dead? Was Jesus God in human form? But Jesus came from a woman's body, so he couldn't be completely pure, and God must be totally pure—this was a real argument! Mary's vagina kept Jesus from being spiritually clean enough to be God. Early Christians even devised a two-thirds compromise to quell divisions, allowing Jesus to be part human and part God.

Resurrection is complicated. I kept asking my doctors, when will I be back to normal? And they would talk about which milestones I needed to pass before I could get a job, live independently, do the regular things that my peers were doing. But that wasn't my question; I wanted to go back to who I was before the Big Depression. I wanted to be optimistic and brave again. I wanted to go back to being a happy, popular college student. Sure, I had been anxious, but I hid it well. I wanted to move back into the big yellow house just off campus, with my six best friends. I wanted senior year road trips and keg parties. I wanted everything back that I had lost. A big rewind to before.

Finally, my no-nonsense therapist Donna said, "What you thought was normal is over. You are different now. Not worse, but different. Say goodbye to the happy but naïve Kate. This is normal now."

As much as it sucked, she was right. There was no total resurrection. I couldn't go back. And as much as I hate to keep comparing myself to Jesus—cause how much more conceited can I get?—I can't help but think of how it would feel to wake up, in spirit and maybe in body, three days after crucifixion. His friends have fled. He was treated cruelly by not only government officials but also everyday people, people he never met, who jeered at him as he carried his cross to Golgotha. On the cross he cried out to God and heard—what? Anything? Did he cry for God and, like me, feel only abandonment and despair? After all of it—the friends fleeing, the torture, the jeering strangers, the agonizing death, and finally calling for God and hearing nothing but his own shallow, pain-filled breath—did he even want to be resurrected? I picture Jesus waking up in the tomb and having mixed thoughts. Or even thinking, "Damn it, not this again."

Because resurrection didn't mean rewinding life back to before the moment before everything went wrong. Jesus couldn't go back to his "greatest hits" and begin there. He couldn't go back to feeding 5,000 people with a few fish and loaves, or walking on water, or bringing his buddy Lazarus back to life. He had to begin from the present moment. A moment in a cold, dark tomb just outside the town where he was murdered. And I had to begin from the present as well.

After my year of mental illness, I was ragged. Pre–nervous breakdown, I had applied for internships in New York City, San Francisco, even Paris, but gave up on all of those when I couldn't even stop crying long enough to get through a phone interview. I was working very, very hard to just stay out of the hospital's psych ward; I spent my days at group therapy and individual therapy and the doctor's office for medication adjustments. I wasn't ready to move out of my childhood bedroom, much less to Paris. Somehow, through the incredible kindness of my professors, I was able to make up just enough classwork to pass my classes and graduate from college. I should have been grateful, but I was so jealous of my peers moving to new places, starting new jobs. A shockingly high number were getting married and pregnant, maybe not in that order. I wanted to be a real adult too. I needed to feel like more than just a psych patient, even though it took 99 percent of my energy to stay sane. I wanted a job.

The problem was that I thought I was cool. I mean, sure, I had had a nervous breakdown in the middle of my senior year of college. And sure, I was still living at home with my parents, who bugged me to go to bed earlier and eat whole grains. And my antidepressants gave me tremors when I got nervous. But I had this idea that I was a cool girl, like Chloe Sevigny or Liz Phair, artsy and punk. Through high school and college, I listened to bands the popular kids had never heard of and made weird outfits out of thrift store finds. I had blue hair decades before everyone had blue hair; I wore too much eyeliner; I talked about the patriarchy and refused to shave my legs and pits. My boyfriend Drew looked like Eddie Vedder, with long, wild curls and flannel shirts over corduroy shorts. Surely that counted for something. I was a wreck, but I still looked kind of cool.

I DJed in college (see Cool Girl, above), playing an alternative show in the evenings: lots of Garbage, the Afghan Wigs, Eels, PJ Harvey. I made sardonic remarks about current events and quoted *Rolling Stone* (never *Spin*) magazine. So, post grad, with my theater degree in hand, I applied to every radio station in my hometown for a DJ job. I interviewed at the classical music station, an interview I blew by mispronouncing Debussy (FYI, it's not De-BUS-e). I blew an interview at the local rap station by being unable to name any rap songs besides those by MC Hammer (my musical taste was problematically Caucasian oriented). But I nailed my interview at the pop station because they produced a lot of advertising in-house and I have the perfect voice for enthusing about mattress liquidation sales and buying fake diamond earrings for Mother's Day. You need a perky voice-over with a Midwestern accent? I'm your woman.

My enthusiasm for the job was short lived. First, I couldn't choose the music—there was a set list for every hour, and I just hit play. No switching out songs, no changing the order. There was plenty of Britney Spears, Matchbox Twenty, and Creed. Pure hell. And if you are thinking, "How bad could it be? It's just cheesy music," it was the same cheesy songs every hour, for six hours at a time. And then there was the banter—I couldn't get it right. The boss said to keep it happy and light, but I said the word "tunes," which was too old-fashioned, when I was supposed to say "track." I wasn't excited enough about new "tracks," and I didn't use popular slang words.

The station manager decided that we all needed to take on young-person personas from pop culture. I was assigned the name Joie and instructed to act just like Joey, the character on the popular teen drama series *Dawson's Creek* played by Katie Holmes. Be the girl next door, the station manager said. Be the pretty virgin who doesn't know she is hot, the squeaky-clean girl all the boys want to seduce.

It was gross, a middle-aged man saddling the female DJs with sweet-but-hot identities while the male DJs were instructed to be raunchy, loud, frat-boy types. We were encouraged to laugh at the guys' jokes but not make our own, and to never, ever make fun of them on air. This was the broadcasting cardinal sin: mocking a man. All the DJs were required to do remote broadcasts, occasions where we were live on-air from an exciting event like the opening of a used-car dealership. While were we there, our fake TV-inspired personas had to be flawless. The nice-no-matter-what piece was the most painful to enact. Joie was supposed to be happy to talk to anyone, even leering guys whose language was thick with innuendo. But that innuendo had to go over Joie's head—she was the innocent virgin. So while a lot of the guys who approached us at the remote broadcasts deserved a kick in the balls, we had to be sweet, while the male DJs made fart jokes and said "that's what she said" over and over.

It was the broadcasting equivalent of working at Hooters, but for minimum wage. My goal was to work there a few years and then try to get a job in public radio, but I didn't even make it three months. Half of my frustration came from trying to appear normal when I was having anxiety attacks, trying to be cool while medication side effects made me nauseous. I was so much better than a few months before, but I was far from back to normal. I hardly remembered normal, except that once I had been a cool girl with dreams of overthrowing the patriarchy and now I was getting paid to laugh at guys' jokes and never make my own. I didn't know who I was, but I was sure Joie wasn't her. I gave my two weeks' notice and stopped showing up after one. I wasn't Joie, so I didn't have to be nice.

14.

Great Jobs I Got
Fired From

Terrible radio station job behind me, I started
looking for another new beginning. The first resurrection
hadn't worked out; could I get a do-over? I was still attempting to be a normal young adult while spending most of my
energy trying not to cry in public. Depression and anxiety
were my closest and most constant companions. Still, I
managed to fake being competent through two interviews
and was hired at a regional theater company in Cincinnati.
This meant I got to move out of my parents' house, which
was both scary for them (I had been suicidal so recently—
could they really trust that I was well enough to get by
without them?) and a relief (empty nest party!).

I got an apartment with Drew and two of his friends,
two floors of a divided-up old house. It was an elegant but

poorly maintained place with hardwood floors, two fire-places, and lots of roaches. Drew and I got to share a bedroom for the first time, which seemed very sophisticated, even more so because our moms didn't like it (living in sin and all). Mike, Drew's childhood best friend, had a room that, like ours, was in the basement and always smelled damp and moldy. Jodi lived upstairs. She and Drew worked together at a hippie nonprofit that canvassed door to door asking for money for environmental organizations, and they complained a lot about The Man. Jodi taught me about organic food; it's hard to believe now, but I didn't know anything about pesticides, herbicides, or why the moldy, misshapen oranges at the food co-op were better than the perfectly round, gorgeously bright oranges at the regular grocery. Jodi also stored stashes of pot all over the house, constantly forgetting where she had left them and searching behind books and under couch cushions. She was my first sexually liberated friend, having no-strings sex with many a dreadlocked white guy on the slanted roof outside her bedroom window.

Our house became famous for this sex display, which Jodi was proud of, and for Jodi's stinky old cat that growled at everyone. It was that kind of a neighborhood, college students living in run-down rentals with couches on the porch, artists and activists drawn to the coffeehouse culture, the hole-in-the-wall bars with live music every night. I thought it was bohemian and felt like I was in *Rent*. There

STUBBORN GRACE

was Ethiopian food, two vegetarian restaurants, and an underground coffee shop where people smoked inside and the staff were really mean. At twenty-two, fresh out of the mental ward and living with my Eddie Vedder–hot boyfriend, it was heaven. Heaven without God, since I was still very angry about feeling ditched by God.

My job was in the box office at the regional theater. The work itself was dull—sell tickets, exchange tickets, reprint tickets—but it was cool-adjacent. Every day, weird things were carried past the box office—a pair of giant wolf heads, an eight-foot-wide replica of a duck's nest, a wall of glass painted to look like an aquarium tank full of fish. Actors were always around, flirting and being supernaturally attractive. They would bring us snacks, flowers, all sorts of little things to butter us up so they could get good seats for family and friends coming to see them in productions. In the ticket office, we got free tickets to every show in town, because the smaller theater companies wanted the directors and producers at our big theater to see them perform and hopefully whisk them from the storefront stage to the big leagues. But the directors and producers never wanted to go, so the tickets went to us, and every week I saw two or three performances. It was a great education because I had decided to put my theater degree to good use and become a director. Now, only a person naïve enough to major in theater thinks it's that simple, but I started calling myself a director and managed to talk my way into some directing

139

jobs around town in tiny theaters. I'm not sure the productions were memorable to anyone but me, but I had fun working on them, and earned all of two or three hundred dollars for my six weeks of evening work.

On the outside, my life was going terrifically: Drew was a wonderfully kind, fun boyfriend. We had friends who we met up with every weekend at Cody's, a local bar with live music and sweet potato fries (the crazy foods they have in the big city!), and I worked in the box office all day and directed plays at night. Our apartment was often full of Drew's activist friends, and Mike was always stirring some hearty vegan goulash on the stove. My theater friends were loud and creative and generous with what little they had. I was happy sometimes. But most of my energy was still going to controlling my anxiety and depression. It was so hard to keep up a façade of normality. I would sneak away from a big party to cry in the bathroom for fifteen minutes, then wash my face and rejoin the crowd. I would keep my nervousness hidden all morning and then have a panic attack on my lunch break.

The weirdest thing about my life was how quickly I stopped being a religious person. I grew up going to church, to vacation Bible school, to church camp. My friends, and nearly all my peers, were churchgoers. During lunch at school we talked about faith the same way we talked about the prom—it was a fact. Jesus was real, God was watching over us. I went to a Christian college and continued spending 99 percent of my time with Christians who were active in church life.

My diaries from elementary school are full of statements like, "I am so glad that God brought Rebecca to my class so we can be friends—God is always so good to me." It was a very simple version of faith, completely normal for that age. I thought that if I behaved and did the things my Sunday school teachers said God wanted done, I would be rewarded with friends like Rebecca. It was typical Mythic-Literal faith stage stuff. In high school, I wrote about how worried I was that God was trying to tell me what to study in college, which career to choose, but I couldn't hear the messages. Should I read the Bible more often? Was I praying wrong? I was desperate to follow God's plan, but first I needed to know what that plan was.

Post Big Depression, I cut God out of my life the way I used to cut off boys who dumped me: destroy any photos of them, don't call them, don't ever let yourself think about them. I was in a big snit with God. For the first time in my life, I wasn't praying multiple times a day. I wasn't reading the Bible. Most significantly, I wasn't planning my life around trying to serve God. Every big life decision had been made with the question, "What is best for the world that God created? How could I best serve?" I didn't want to be a missionary or anything evangelical, but I did want a future that involved making the world easier for people who were suffering. Now, post breakdown, after dumping God, I felt unmoored. It was, frankly, very lonely. I realized that I had spent most of my life in a dialogue with God and then severed that connection. Now how should I navigate?

After about a year in the box office, I was fired. My work wasn't good: my accounts never balanced, I forgot to do routine things, customers could tell I was distracted. How, my boss wondered, could someone with a college degree have so much trouble with such simple tasks? This was the first great job I was fired from. It wasn't that I loved selling tickets, but it was wonderfully fun to be a part of a large, well-funded and well-managed theater company. My job wasn't creative, but there were so many creative jobs I could have been promoted into if I had been successful in the box office. It was my first full-time job, and while it didn't pay well, it paid enough to go out to eat once in a while before one of the many free productions I got to go to because of the job. I thought I would work there for years and years, maybe my whole life, getting promoted into more and more creative roles. But I wasn't keeping up the façade of Not Mentally Ill as well as I had hoped.

My boss was right: I was distracted. I screwed up over and over. I was managing my mental illnesses and a lot of pharmaceutical side effects, and that took too much effort for me to also focus on balancing my accounts. My boss didn't know all I was coping with, and I don't blame him for firing me. I was doing the best I could, and it wasn't good enough. It was terrifying. Being fired made me doubt all the progress I had made—would I end up like Sharon after all? I was trying so hard to live a normal life. Every waking moment took a tremendous amount of effort to be normal— and still I failed? I was so tired. I didn't want to die but wondered if suicide was inevitable when I couldn't seem to make life work. Since I had dumped God, I wasn't worried about Hell anymore. I figured death meant total oblivion. It didn't sound so bad.

At some point during a psych hospitalization, a group therapist had said maybe I should try living in a group home. At first I was excited because I thought he meant a commune. A group home where we would grow our own vegetables and cook together and paint protest banners in the living room sounded excellent. But no, he clarified that he meant a group home for adults who can't live independently. A group home for people with mental illness. A house with a social worker checking in on me and lots of rules about when I could come and go, lots of life supervision. Fuck that, I thought. I don't need another group of people telling me what to do. Fuck that—I was backpacking through Europe a year ago, I slept on the stairs of a cathedral, I flirted in Italian, I made sense of French train timetables. I am not living in a fucking group home with some do-gooder babysitter making sure I eat my vegetables, making sure I take the bus to whatever low-skilled job they set up for me. But now, fired, depressed, exhausted, I wondered, if it was between a group home or moving back in with Mom and

Dad, which would I choose? At least Mom and Dad didn't talk to me in the condescending social-worker voice I heard at the hospital.

I might have given up and moved back in with my parents, resigned to being too crazy to live independently, if it hadn't been for Drew. I was crying on our front porch when he got home, which wasn't unusual. Depressed people cry a lot. But when I told him I had been fired, I thought he would agree that I should probably move back home. Instead, he was incensed on my behalf. He said they must be idiots to let me go and that it was just one job—a job I wasn't really suited for anyway, being mostly math, which I hated. He convinced me that this was a minor setback, not an indication that I couldn't make it living on my own. It was just one dumb job, and I could find another.

How lucky was I to have someone who was so good at loving me? I was a mess—crying constantly, having tremors from my meds. I never cooked or cleaned (not because of mental illness, though, I'm just lazy). I was fixated on suicide and felt gross most of the time from medication side effects. Drew was healthy, so handsome that women flirted with him right in front of me, and smart. He brought me flowers and made me oatmeal with cinnamon every morning. It was impossible to feel like a loser when someone like Drew wanted to be with me. I held it close to my chest, like precious evidence: Drew loves me and he is really smart, so

I must be lovable. I can do this. It is really hard, but I can keep going.

I thought about what my therapist Donna had said when I told her I was moving out of my parents' house. She said I should get a job at a coffee shop, a bookstore, maybe a movie theater that plays independent films. But nothing I wanted to turn into a career, she said, for five or ten years. You need to think about how you are going to spend your energy, and choose to spend it on healing your mind, on creating a balanced, healthy life, not on learning a complex job or trying to get promoted. She wanted me to give myself five or ten years to just figure out how to be happy, even with depression and anxiety disorders.

It was really good advice that I immediately ignored. My ego took a big hit when I had to drop out of school, go into the hospital, and then get rejected by my former friends. Pre-depression, I was focused on graduating with honors and landing a fancy internship, and instead I was lucky to graduate at all. My ego wanted an important job, something I could brag about. A job to prove I wasn't a crazy loser. A low-key, low-prestige job was just what my soul needed, but my ego was louder than my desire for well-being. So I got a job at an abortion clinic.

A friend of Drew's, a super-cool woman our age who somehow already had her shit together, got me an interview for a patient advocate position. If you have never lived in southern Ohio, first, I am so sorry. Second, it's conservative. Conservative in a Christian fundamentalist way. Conservative in a "Mom, I can't go to Young Life (a cultish Bible study group for Christian youth) tonight because my Christian Athletes for Christ (Bible thumpers who are also good at soccer) meeting is right after my True Love Waits (cultish abstinence-only group for Christian youth) pizza party." So my interview at the abortion clinic first involved finding it; it was hidden away on a side street, behind a strip mall, with huge shade trees blocking the sign. This low profile was to protect patients and stick it to protestors: sure, they had the constitutional right to come harass people outside the clinic, but they weren't getting any extra attention from bystanders this far off the main drag.

The second part of the interview was to scare the bejesus out of me with horror stories about the violence that clinic staff faced just by coming to work. The center had a bomb threat at least once a week. While I was there, the police were called because a man was outside with a gun, threatening to shoot his former girlfriend, who was inside. The building had no windows, and the double doors were bulletproof glass. 911 was on speed dial. The clinic's director listed all these terrifying incidents and more, so I knew what I was getting into by working there. Was it worth it to me? Did I want the job badly enough to face the harassment in the parking lot every day, the bomb threats, the abusive boyfriends trying to get inside? Yes, I said. Yes—but inside I knew it was not because I was noble but because I was stubborn.

Did these forced-birth assholes really think they were going to keep me from getting a job that not only paid two dollars over minimum wage but also had insane bragging rights? Talk about feminist credibility. "Sure," the broken pieces of my ego called out, "sure, threaten to blow up the place—I almost died at my own hand, you think you're going to scare me?" And yes, I believe in reproductive freedom, and yes, I wanted to help people get the health services that every human is entitled to receive. But also, boy was I excited to tell people about my super-feminist new job.

I went into it for the wrong reasons, so don't feel too bad that I got fired after only two weeks. Two weeks! At least I lasted a year at the theater. The problem was crying, mostly, but also sleeping. I cried so much at work. It was hard not to—women came in to have abortions for a lot of reasons, many of them related to rape and incest. In two weeks, I spoke with three teenage girls raped by stepfathers. There were college students who just had one (roofied) drink at a party and woke up the next morning naked, pregnant, and with no memory of who, what, or how many. Plus, so many women who would have continued the pregnancy but couldn't leave their low-paying service job, couldn't afford childcare, who had to sell their TV, their car, and their couch just to pay for the abortion.

Very few men entered the clinic. Boyfriends, husbands, hook-ups—all mysteriously absent, despite most pregnancies coming from sex with a man. Every day there was a depressing lack of male support in the waiting room. There were calls from men, calls asking if a particular woman was there. Of course, we didn't say, as medical care is confidential. But lots of men on the phone trying to threaten us into saying if their wife, girlfriend, or sister was getting an abortion. Trying to control the body of a woman he claimed to love.

There was some joy in the clinic. In the postprocedure recovery room, where patients sat sipping juice while nurses checked vital signs, there was palpable relief. Nearly every person expressed a version of "Was that it? That wasn't so bad!" Laughing together, women realized that this was a blip on the radar of their life, not the defining story. Not the moment that ruined everything.

The patients I worried about the most were the ones I never met. Several times a day, a person would call who was underage. In Ohio, a girl under eighteen has to have parental permission to have an abortion, making the procedure impossible for many girls from hyperreligious families. The conversations were heart-wrenching. A girl would call; we would confirm that she needed parental permission; she would tell us about how her mom was an addict and she didn't know her dad, that she lived on the streets or with a foster family who would kick her out when they found out she was pregnant. This was a common, terrible situation: parents expelling kids from home for being pregnant but also refusing permission to get an abortion on religious grounds. Because God is okay with you kicking out your kid, pretty much guaranteeing they will be homeless, won't be able to graduate from high school, might end up sex trafficked—but not okay with you letting her abort an embryo? It was hell telling girls that we couldn't make an exception for them so they could end their pregnancy, finish high school, and have a chance at a happy life. I cried and cried while telling girls we would be shut down if we let them exercise their own self-determination, if we honored their bodily autonomy. If a girl is old enough to become pregnant, she is old enough to determine if she wants to be pregnant. But in many states, girls are forced to be parents before they are old enough to choose to get an abortion.

Occasionally, these situations ended happily. One pregnant teenager wept as I told her that she needed parental permission for her procedure. "They'll kill me," she cried. I encouraged her to tell them in the presence of a trusted adult, an aunt or a teacher. "I just can't, they'll kill me." Too often, this isn't an exaggeration—if you want to be really depressed, do an internet search for how often girls are killed by parents (or boyfriends) for being pregnant. But this girl was lucky—a few days later she came to the clinic, signed parental permission form in hand, with one parent on either side of her. They kept their arms around her as we checked her in, her dad made corny jokes as he paid for the procedure, and they sat laughing over magazines in the waiting room, talking about her going to volleyball camp, discussing which colleges she might apply to. Her abortion went normally, as they usually do; it is a relatively minor medical procedure. On their way out that afternoon, they discussed lunch options and that, yes, she had to go back to school the next day.

That was a rare positive occasion. Patients told me their stories as I explained the procedure and what to expect. By Ohio law, I had to offer them a packet of materials on adoption that included incorrect fetal pictures, images provided by an anti-choice organization that lied about when developments occurred in the timeline of pregnancy. Images of a fetus showed distinct humanlike characteristics that were strictly artistic license. The packet was rife with misinformation, and it seemed to make patients think they had to justify their choice to have an abortion to me, which they did not. I honor every person's bodily autonomy, and I know that scientifically an embryo is less "alive" than a gnat. But they shared their stories, and I frequently wept.

I know now that a more appropriate reaction would be to empathize and to emphasize hope. To focus on the new beginning they would have when they were no longer pregnant. But I was young, and depressed, and so I cried with patients. Often they would end up comforting me, which was the opposite of the clinic's intention. Often I had to take breaks afterward to calm down, which meant longer wait times for patients who just wanted to get on with their lives.

Even worse, sometimes I feel asleep while counseling patients. That didn't go over well with management. Since I was crying too much at work, I increased my antidepressant medication, which made me sleepy. So, instead of weeping, I dozed off. That is what finally caused the manager to fire me. I spent an hour trying to talk her out of it, but deep down, I knew she was right. Yes, the work meant a great deal to me. It was the most important work I had ever done, perhaps the most important work I have ever done. And I desperately wanted to do a good job because the patients were important to me. But I wasn't healthy enough to do a decent job. Even when I wasn't crying or dozing off, I was foggy-headed from medication. I wasn't sleeping well because I couldn't stop thinking about patients who had been raped, molested, kicked out. I couldn't separate my work life from my private life, so I just worried and cried constantly.

It was the opposite of the kind of job Donna the therapist had recommended. The emotional intensity, the bomb threats, the constant vigilance—today I am surprised it didn't send me back to thinking about suicide. Was my ego trying to kill me? Was having a job I could brag about this important? No. Time to forget about great jobs and focus on finding something meaningless to fill my days, so I could work on my well-being.

15.

The Patriarchy Always Knocks Twice

WHILE I WORKED at the abortion clinic, I was directing a play in the evening at a small theater company. The theater was semiprofessional, which meant that I got paid just enough to cover my gas. The comedy had an all-female cast of hilarious performers who were fun to work with. The show opened the week after I got fired, and unlike my employment situation, it was a huge success. It was the top-selling production in the theater company's history and ran for two extra weeks. At the cast party, after the last show, the artistic director told me which plays had been selected for the next season and told me I could have my choice of them to direct.

The plays selected by management to be performed by theater companies was something I moaned and groaned about a lot. I was young and idealistic; I wanted to direct plays about the AIDS crisis and surviving incest and racial biases—really happy topics. But artistic directors, concerned about staying financially afloat, chose plays that would sell tickets. Musicals, comedies, anything by Neil Simon; those shows played over and over, year after year. I thought I was way too cool to direct that popular fluff. I didn't want people to actually enjoy going to the theater; I wanted it to change their outlook, to make them rebel and overthrow the heteronormative paradigm. So I was excited when the artistic director told me that there was a Sam Shepard play in the next season.

I told him that was my pick, I'd take the Sam Shepard, please, and he started to laugh. He laughed so hard he started coughing. "A woman can't direct Sam Shepard!"

It felt impossible that he was really that sexist, so I asked what was so funny. Was this some kind of inside joke and I was missing the punch line? The artistic director was a young, hip guy, a person of color. He didn't really mean that my lady parts meant no directing Sam Shepard?

But he did. He explained that Sam Shepard focused on men—their anger, their struggles with masculinity, with nurturing relationships and still being manly. I countered that, having spent my whole life in a world focused on men, I could certainly empathize with their struggles. And it isn't like all men are 100-percent masculinity and women 100-percent femininity. I have been told plenty of times that I am too much of a guy: too loud, too bossy, too powerful. We are all a mix of ideas about gender and identity, not just male or female.

He just said "Yeah, no. No woman can direct Shepard. Pick something else."

This should have been an incredible night of celebration: I directed the longest running show in the company's history. I was on my way to a raucous cast party that would probably go until dawn. And yet, standing in the dark theater, hand on the doorknob, I knew I wouldn't be coming back. Sure, I wasn't experienced enough to be choosy about the theaters I would work with. Sure, I could choose any other show in the next season. But I walked away.

Directing a play is an enormous investment of time, energy, and emotion. At the semiprofessional level, there is very little financial compensation. I needed to know that I was devoting myself to a project with people whom I could respect and who respected me. I am sure the artistic director would have claimed to respect me, but it was no matter—I lost my respect for him that evening. Professionally, it wasn't the right choice. I struggled to get other gigs of that caliber, considering how little experience I had. But I had tried to go along with misogyny at the radio station. I was quiet about sexism there because I wanted to get enough experience to get a position somewhere better. I quickly lost respect for my coworkers and even myself. I didn't want to set a standard, especially this early in my adult life, of being ethically malleable in order to get ahead professionally. If I bent my own rules once, twice, when would I know to stop? In my anger at God, I had left faith behind, but not a sense of right and wrong behavior.

My sense of morality was called into question a few months later. I took Donna's advice and got a job in a coffee shop, not one of the cool ones with odd music playing too loud and tattooed baristas but a mall food court place where a friend worked. It was an easy and surprisingly satisfying job. All of my tasks were manageable, and I could see the results of my work: I washed a stack of dishes and saw that the kitchen was decluttered. I restocked the straws and saw that the caddy was neat and full. The mindlessness was pleasant, especially with directing gigs taking up my concentration in the evening.

I had one coworker, John, who made me nervous. He was my age and quite handsome and charming—but there was something underneath his charm that made me uncomfortable. I began to see how he manipulated the women on the staff, talking them into doing the more onerous tasks while he stood at the front counter and flirted with customers. He frequently bragged about being pre-med, a future cardiologist, but when I asked him which classes he was taking specifically, he caged around before admitting that he was taking this quarter off from the community college.

Then a young woman came in, his former girlfriend, with his baby. She asked him if he had taken his GED yet, and he shot her a deadly glare. She left quickly.

A few days later, John tried to sweet-talk me into mopping the bathroom floor, which was his closing job. I said no, and he flirted some more, but I still refused. I hated the smell of the mop bucket, and anyway, why should I do his work? There were few other employees around when he transformed from flirty to cruel, suddenly screaming, "Why do you have to be such a stubborn dyke bitch?" and slapping me hard across the face. Tears rose to my eyes, but fury pushed them back down, and I reached for the phone to call our manager at home.

The other employee, also a young man, an awkward, pimply guy who adored John, hung up the phone and told me to get over it, that he would mop the floor. He said to quit egging John on. I told him that John didn't get to slap me and picked up the phone again. John said, "I'm going to fucking kill you, bitch," and I walked out.

I was absolutely terrified. It was late in the evening, and the mall was closing. I had to walk a few blocks to the bus stop and then wait for the bus to arrive. The whole time I looked around me, looked all around me, waiting for John to attack. I didn't see him, and finally I got home and locked the deadbolt behind me. I collapsed, crying on the floor, and finally called the local police to report my assault.

I would love to report that the police were helpful and sympathetic, as were my manager and coworkers. Unfortunately, that wasn't the case. The police said that while a slap in the face was technically an assault, it wasn't enough for them to write up a report. They refused to take any action, not even talking to the coworker who witnessed the event or to John. I would be shocked if they even wrote down his name. The next day the manager told me he had heard about what had happened and, "since John and I couldn't get along," he would put us on different shifts. "But this better not be a problem with anyone else," he added, along with a big eye roll.

I told him John should be fired. He said, "You know that guy is pre-med? He has a kid to take care of; why would you want to mess his life up?" As if it was my fault. He added, "Bad enough that his ex keeps trying to charge him with bullshit accusations." I could guess those accusations; she had probably been the victim of his violent temper as well.

I quit. It was just a coffee shop job, but it still bothered me: the second time that misogyny had ended an opportunity. I was lucky to be in a position to leave—work in the service industry for any time at all, and you will hear horrible stories of employee abuse: sexual, verbal, and physical. Many people would be stuck working with John for months or even years, mopping floors to appease him. Doing anything to keep him from snapping again.

Throughout my life, I have been fortunate to have lots of experiences working with smart, kind people. And I have occasionally worked with men who hate women. Not who hate just me or who are just sexist—they feel a deep disdain for all women. John was the first, but not the last. Woman-haters are in the arts, in seminaries, and in churches. I have learned to listen to my instincts when I feel that a man is hiding behind charm.

My two encounters with misogynists set me back in emotional health. After those incidents, I felt out of control of my life. I had worked hard and been successful, and still my work was derailed. Anger coursed through me, and I felt that my efforts were futile. What difference did it make if I was smart, or talented, or a good Christian, or even a nice person? Did any of it matter at all? I wanted to stop caring. If I didn't care, then it wouldn't matter if I succeeded or failed.

During college, I had the occasional drink, and now and then smoked some pot. I liked the feeling of loose limbs that came with being a little intoxicated. Not out of control, but less anxious. Now I began to drink more often, and I didn't stop after one or two cocktails. I wasn't drinking to feel relaxed; I was drinking to get drunk. I got high so I could forget about my Big Depression and getting fired. I wanted to feel like someone else, someone who truly didn't care about repercussions.

I was also having difficulty affording health care. After I got fired from my box office position, I lost my health insurance. I paid out of pocket for visits to the psychiatrist, $180 per session (consider that my rent at the time was only $240 a month). I was supposed to go every month but went twice a year; it was too expensive. I couldn't afford to buy monthly doses of my prescriptions, so I went to the pharmacy every week or so, when I had scraped together tips or gotten a birthday check, to get a few days' worth of pills. The medications added up to around $500 a month. I missed a lot of doses because of lack of funds. While weekly therapy sessions had done me a tremendous amount of good, they were impossible to afford, and I stopped going altogether.

With irregular medication usage, no money for therapy, and certainly no money for extras like a yoga class or gym membership, my mood nosedived. I began to drink too much when I was out with my actor friends and a few times drove home drunk. Twice I remember driving to work in the morning and realizing that I was probably still too drunk to be driving. I took so many stupid risks and feel lucky I never hurt anyone. I did wake up one day to dents all along one side of my car—maybe someone sideswiped me and I was too drunk to notice? Maybe I sideswiped someone and was too drunk to notice?

It hurts to remember how selfish I was during this time, getting so drunk that Drew worried about me. He said that he wondered how to keep me safe when I seemed so bent on destroying myself. At that moment I realized he was right:

I was trying to destroy myself. My life just hurt too much. I couldn't bear feeling so sad and anxious. I couldn't bear the losses or the first few years of my adult life—being fired from the box office and the abortion clinic, quitting the directing gig and the coffee shop. The trauma of my hospitalizations and Sharon's death and all the horrible stories at the abortion clinic and getting slapped by my coworker and discounted by the police. It was too much.

Drew started to cry, and I realized that I needed to choose: either life or death. Either quit being reckless and hiding from reality with intoxication or just commit suicide. Wasn't that what I was edging toward, anyway? Why else choose to drive drunk, if not because I hoped it would kill me?

I decided I wanted to live. I had this memory of the first sunny day after Sharon ended her life. She died during the bleakest part of winter, when it was cloudy for weeks and bitterly cold. The snow was piled high on the sides of the road, and it was filthy with exhaust and grime. Then, finally, the sun came out. The snow melted. The sky was that hopeful bright blue that promises spring will come. And I couldn't stop thinking that if Sharon had seen this sky, felt this soft sunshine on her skin, she wouldn't have done it. She wouldn't have ended her life. Not that the sun was enough—I understood how awful depression felt, the physical agony of it, the crushing hopelessness. But if she had seen the sun, she would have believed that it would end.

Just as winter had to eventually end, so did depression. The blue sky wouldn't heal her and the sun wouldn't cure her, but they would give her enough hope to hold on until the pharmaceuticals started to work.

I didn't want to die and miss the next sunny day. Or the next thrilling thunderstorm, with lightning arcing across the sky before nosediving into a momentarily lit-up cornfield. The next Christmas morning, opening presents in my pajamas with my parents and brother. The first watermelon of the season. My medications dampened my sexual response, but I heard from friends about reality-shattering orgasms, and I wanted to live long enough to experience those too.

I talked through all these thoughts with Drew. He promised to remind me of them if I got too depressed to remember all the reasons I wanted to live. We fell asleep in each other's arms, another miraculously sweet feeling worth holding on for. And we decided to get married.

16.

Good Choices, Bad Reasons

BAD REASONS to get married:

1. Codependence. I am afraid if Drew isn't around to take care of me, I might go back into the hospital, have to live in a group home, or decide to end my life.
2. Parental concerns. Our moms are mad that we are living together, so if we get married, they will relax.
3. Fear of loss. I lost my college friends and then God because of my mental illness. I didn't want anyone else disappearing on me.
4. Anchoring. I wanted to attach myself to a normal person who would make me feel rooted

again. So much of the time, I felt unreal. I was anxious in situations in which there was no need to be anxious. I cried when life was going fine. I felt like an observer floating on the outside of everyone else's reality, trying to figure out how they kept their emotions in check, managed not to get fired, didn't cry every few hours. Drew was good at normal life. Anchored to him, I would learn how to be normal.

5. Everyone else is doing it. We went to college in a little town where lots of our friends got married the summer after graduation. Marriage would prove we were as grown up as they were; we loved each other as much as they did.

Please don't get the wrong idea—we were completely in love. Drew was a gentle, kind, and generous boyfriend. He was the funniest and smartest person I knew. It was impossible to imagine loving anyone more than I loved him. But the truth is, I used him. I needed someone to take care of me. I wanted him to protect me from my scary emotions, to defend me from life's unfairness. So I asked him to marry me so that he would always have to help me.

We got married a few months later, in his aunt and uncle's soybean field. A friend read a Kahlil Gibran poem; another sang an Indigo Girls song. Looking at pictures of that day, I can see that I was completely, entirely happy, in every cell of my body. I think Drew was too. We were very young, very unsure of the future, and very willing to cling to each other as we tried to make it through. We were so broke that we didn't even have money for a honeymoon, so we got married on Saturday and went back to work on Monday. But all day at work, customers commented on my glow.

17.

Stealing Junk

MARRIAGE DID CALM DOWN my anxiety, or at least the anxiety was overridden by all the glowing romance of being newly married. Drew and I spent a lot of time looking into each other's eyes, kissing on street corners, and writing each other love notes on the backs of student loan bills. We had plenty of debt, plenty of overdue notices, and not nearly enough money, which we tried not to think about while singing emo love songs to each other. But eventually, the worry ate away at my happiness. I had stomachaches, and my heart raced thinking about how we were going to pay our bills.

I worked in the kind of coffeeshop for which the word *twee* was invented. It had passed by cute and run into syrupy sweetness. It was a tiny, old-fashioned kind of building on a busy corner, shaped like a slice of cake. The same customers came in most days, and we served them homemade scones and hot herbal tea for a significant markup. The shop was in an affluent neighborhood, and it amazed me how much people would pay for coffee and baked goods. Starbucks hadn't come to town yet, and the shop owner was ahead of the game on coffee as a luxury purchase, coffee as a way to show off wealth. After all, if you could carry around a $5 latte with the coffeeshop name printed in bold on the cup, what couldn't you afford? Most people back then made coffee at home, for a nickel or so a cup. But those disposable coffee cups were a status symbol, a sign you had money to waste.

There was nothing wrong with the job, except that the boss was always grouchy and it paid minimum wage in a neighborhood where teenagers drove BMWs to private day schools. The comparison chafed. Sure, I had a fancy liberal arts college degree, and I was white and young and looked healthy—those were the reasons I got to work in a fancy coffee shop and not in a fast food joint. I had barrels of privilege compared to people of color in the strictly segregated city of Cincinnati. All the women—and it was all women, and all white women—who worked at the coffee shop had degrees (some advanced degrees), and we were all artistic in some way or another—painters, potters, poets. We could all discuss articles in the *New Yorker* and relate, or pretend to relate, when customers came in to moan about how long renovations were taking at their vacation house at Hilton Head. We were hired because we made rich people feel comfortable. They weren't challenged by our skin color, and they didn't have to feel bad about educational disparities because we had gone to college.

The disparity in wealth did chafe though. It was irritating to be tipped fifty cents by a woman in Prada spending forty-five dollars on baked goods to take to her book club. Trying to manage my anxiety and crying jags, I got in the habit of volunteering to go down to the basement to get items that needed to be restocked. In that dark and damp, I could sit for a moment on the crates of coffee beans and take deep breaths. And it was while sitting down there that I first stole.

I'm not proud of this stealing, just like I feel awful when I think about drinking and driving. But it was a strange manifestation of my anxiety. Once I stole for the first time, taking a tin of green tea, which I didn't even drink, I couldn't seem to stop. A few times a week, I was sent to the basement to get more coffee filters or cup lids, and I would grab something random from the stock shelves and jam it into my bookbag. All of the staff's coats, scarves, and bags were on hooks in the basement, so it was easy to jam small things into pockets or packs.

It was an odd compulsion, one I had never had before. I didn't steal candy from the gas station when I was little, like some kids did; I didn't ever feel the desire. I'm not sure it had even occurred to me. But when I started to feel panicky, I would sneak off to steal some worthless item.

Decorative tea tins, mugs with corny sayings—stealing junk made me feel calm. I felt in control.

It wasn't a victimless crime. The store was family owned and operated, and just because the owner was a jerk didn't mean I could steal from him. I felt guilty about it then and now. It was a weird way I comforted myself that also made me feel awful. Compulsions have cropped up here and there in my life—my frantic prayer as a child, this desire to steal. Acting compulsively made me feel better in a moment of panic and despair but did nothing to ease the overall pain of mental illness. It was a dangerous band-aid.

Drew was very uncomfortable with my stealing. He was sure I would get caught, sure that the police would get involved. He didn't understand why I did it. I promised, and failed, to quit half a dozen times. I would swear I would never steal again and have that promise in my head all day. I really didn't think I would steal. And then the anxiety would creep back into my body, slowly rising all day. I would work harder and harder to control the tears trying to escape. And I knew that the only way to control my emotions was to steal something. It was that or start crying and yelling, that or storm out of the coffee shop. So I would swipe something. Then I felt instant relief. A wave of calm running across my body. My mind settled. I could go back to normal.

I wish I had been in therapy at the time. I felt shame at stealing. I crammed my pilfered goods in a high kitchen cabinet and refused to look at them. A therapist could have helped me to find better ways to calm down, to re-center. A therapist could have put a quick end to my thefts with self-soothing techniques. But therapy was far, far outside our budget.

Finally, I accidentally quit that job. I told the owner that I needed to make more money and if I didn't get a raise, I was going to have to seek work elsewhere. I was sure he would agree to pay me more, but perhaps he had noticed items missing, or maybe I just wasn't that valuable of an employee, because he said, "So I'll take this as the first day of your two-week notice," and walked away.

Since Drew had been recently laid off, I had accidentally quit, and our rent was going up, we decided to move a few hours away to Columbus. A friend had offered us a house-sitting job there for the summer. Drew felt like we needed a new start, one that involved less theft and debt. With three months of free housing, we could look for jobs that included health insurance, and I could take my medications regularly again, maybe even go to therapy. With the few things we owned packed in the back of a minivan, we headed east to start life in Ohio's capital city.

18.

Accidentally Stealing

DOES IT COUNT AS THEFT if you don't know you are stealing? I'm guessing yes. Drew and I moved into the house we were watching for the summer, the house of our college friend Virginia's grad school professor. The professor was in Europe for the summer and needed someone to stay at her house and water the elaborate garden in the mornings and evenings. We hadn't met her, as she was already in Europe when we arrived, but Virginia showed us around. She lived nearby, in an apartment with her boyfriend.

It was a very nice house, historic and perfectly maintained, with wide windows and dark paneling on the walls of the formal dining room. There was a hot tub in the formal back garden and a big kitchen full of luxury appliances. Shelves of books lined the walls, but sadly they were all in

German, the second language of the homeowner. It was like having a full-size dollhouse to play in—we loved imagining that we owned the house and had intellectual careers, read in foreign languages, and entertained friends from all over the world. We read through the professor's cookbooks and had joking conversations about whether we should make lamb or lobster for our pretend dinner party with our pretend guests.

It was the first glimpse I had of the kind of adult life I wanted to create. Not so wealthy, perhaps, but intellectual, filled with art and books and colorful plants. I was too young to appreciate the comfortable home created by my parents, with its own art and books and colorful plants. I was still in the stage where I wanted to be different from them. This home, with its advanced age and kitchen appliances that screamed, "I have parties with fancy seated dinners that have ingredients you can't even recognize and wine from countries you can't find on a map," seemed to mock our lentil and brown rice meals and our zine-centered reading.

It was a terrifically comfortable seat from which to get our bearings in our new city. We had a little money saved from selling our furniture and TV before moving, so we lived frugally and spent time looking for jobs that we would enjoy and that would include health benefits. With few bills to worry about and a perfect backyard oasis from which to look at job listings, Drew and I were happy. I was the most relaxed I had felt in a few years, with very little anxiety and no depression or compulsions. We finally felt more hopeful than fearful about the future.

Until we found out we were squatting. About three weeks after we moved in, a neighbor stopped by to introduce herself. She expressed surprise that there were two of us housesitting, but I didn't think anything of it until Virginia showed up the next day in tears. Between sobs, the truth of the situation came out. Virginia had agreed to housesit for her professor this summer. Then she met a great guy and they started dating. Eventually he asked her to move in with him and she said yes. But she didn't want to anger her professor and screw up her grad school grades by bailing on the house-sitting gig, so she asked Drew and me to house-sit for her, assuring us that no, we didn't need to meet the professor in person; she trusted us. And assuring herself that no one would ever catch on.

Virginia had good intentions—she really did want to help Drew and me. She knew how depressed I had been and that we were broke. And love makes us all do dumb things, like bail on commitments. But then the professor called the neighbors to make sure the house sitter was there and taking care of the yard and learned that there wasn't one but two sitters. And neither was the student she knew. So Virginia had to kick us out and move herself in before the professor called the police to have us removed.

It was not the calm summer we had looked forward to having. Suddenly we needed jobs and an apartment right away. Suddenly my anxiety was back and bigger than ever. But since Columbus is a college town, we found an apartment quickly, and Drew found a job. I didn't find a day job, but I did get a directing gig with a small company, starting immediately. Through that gig, I found an office job doing bookkeeping—truly the job I am least suited for. But more important, I found a faith community.

I was really missing church. Growing up, Sunday services were the trunk from which all other life branched out. My church taught me how to be in the world, helped me to discover my values. My ministers taught me critical thinking skills and pushed me to try leadership roles that gave me confidence. Church people were the most important people in my life; my youth group friends are so dear to me I think of them as siblings. At church, I learned about music and poetry, about how artistic beauty lifts a person out of the humdrum everyday and into the realm of the sacred and eternal. I missed all of it. Without Sunday morning services, life seemed to spin around without a hub. There were no big philosophical questions to think about and no one to discuss big ideas with. My friends were people my age, with my interests—none of the cross-generational caring that I grew up with.

I missed church, but I was still bitter. I was still angry with God for not saving me from depression. I was mad at religious people because a handful of loud and proud Christians had abandoned me when I needed them the most. But my definition of God was expanding. After years of vitriol at anything spiritual or religious, I found myself hovering in front of the shop window of the local bookstore, scanning a collection of books about Buddhism. I finally sauntered in and saw a whole section labeled Earth Centered, which I had never heard of but sounded intriguing. I was into plants, I felt at my best in the woods—was I a part of a religious category and not even aware of it? I was finally realizing that faith was much bigger, and more diverse, than I had imagined.

The theater company I was working with rehearsed in a huge historic building that housed many nonprofit groups. One weekend, someone left old paint cans and rags lying around, and a fire started. No one was injured, but we had to move our rehearsals. One actor was a member of the Unitarian Universalist Church just down the street. He arranged for us to meet there.

The building was large and modern, with a round sanctuary at one end. There were a lot of entrances, but the main entrance was well marked, and I walked into a light-filled lobby. Bulletin boards lined the hallway to our borrowed rehearsal space, and thumbtacked to them were flyers for a Buddhist study group, a pagan solstice celebration, and a drop-in "Bible Study for Heretics." There was a huge poster advertising the Religious Coalition for Reproductive Choice, a group I had never heard of. I wasn't used to seeing words like *religious* and *choice* in close proximity. Also surprising was a sign-up sheet to guard a billboard.

"Why are you all babysitting billboards?" I asked my actor friend. He reported that the church bought a billboard that said a person could be religious and support abortion rights. Anti-choice groups and religious fundamentalists kept threatening to destroy the billboard, which had cost the church a lot of money. So pairs of volunteers were keeping watch all night, every night to make sure it wasn't damaged. A long list of people had signed up.

I felt dizzy hearing and seeing all of this. First, it made my longing for a church community so sharp that I nearly cried out. I was so hungry for fellowship, for deep religious and philosophical ideas, and for activism rooted in faith. But I had never heard of Unitarian Universalists, and I didn't want to join another Christian denomination. I couldn't join a church that required me to leave some part of myself at the door—my curiosity about Buddhism and paganism, mainly, but also having depression and anxiety. But they had flyers about Buddhism. . . . I wasn't sure what to think. I felt defensive and afraid; my deep hunger left me vulnerable.

I spent several weeks trying not to think about the congregation and failing. I asked a neighbor if she had heard of Unitarian Universalists and learned she had friends who were UUs and were atheists. "What? Atheists at church? How does that work?" She shrugged.

"They don't believe in God, but they wanted the whole church thing—the community, the kids' program for their toddler, thinking about big questions."

Drew, knowing that thoughts about church were pre-occupying me, said, "Why don't you just go check out a service?" He didn't want to go. Raised Catholic, he never enjoyed worship services or felt like he got anything out of them. He had zero fond memories of church, unless you count that his family always went to the local Frisch's Big Boy for the breakfast buffet afterward. Unlimited bacon—that he believed in. Besides, he was shy, and walking into a big group of new people was his worst nightmare.

On a cold and cloudy winter day, I pulled my car into a visitor's parking spot and looked around. The lot was packed—families were pouring out of minivans, and four elderly ladies wearing bright clothes exited a red Volkswagen Bug the same color as their cherry-red lipstick. There were people my age waving hi to each other and teenage boys roughhousing on the lawn. Most people were white, but not all, and there were same-sex couples holding hands, which was unusual in Ohio at the time. About half the crowd was dressed in jeans and sweaters; the other half was dressier.

I went inside, and a friendly usher waved me toward an empty seat. The sanctuary was nearly full. There were a few hundred people, and a woman and a man in robes sat on the chancel in the front. There was lovely, ethereal flute and piano music coming from two musicians up front as well. The service began, and my vision was clouded by tears, tears that streamed down my face for the entire hour. I don't remember many specifics. There was a children's story acted out with puppets and hymns about nature and justice. The sermon included elements from the Bible and the Koran. My mind was stretched, and my heart was full.

I began to attend every Sunday. It was a big congregation, and I appreciated the anonymity that came with being in a crowd. I loved every service, but I was still leery of church people. I didn't stick around for coffee hour to meet people. I wasn't sure that they would still like me once they knew I was an anxious, depressed mess. On the outside, I looked normal. I had a decent job and enjoyed directing plays at night. But I still had an occasional panic attack.

Church attendance helped with my anxiety, though. The periods of meditation, the soothing music, but most of all the chance to look at life through a bigger lens than my everyday experience. During the service we thought about big ideas, not the everyday worrying about health and paying bills. We talked about life in a way that reminded me I was one of billions, a speck of life flashing for a brief second in time. It helped me see my worries in perspective.

I attended the congregation for about a year before Drew and I decided to move to Cleveland. In that time, I stayed on the periphery, volunteering occasionally to bring food to a workshop or make posters for a pro-choice rally.

But even from my view on the periphery, the church began to change my life. I was grounded in something bigger than myself—a quest for meaning. A desire to make the world more just. And it was okay that I didn't have all the answers (or any of the answers) because this was the kind of church where questions were encouraged. I didn't know what the future would hold, but I knew Unitarian Universalism would always be a part of my life.

19.

Two Pink Lines

WHEN THE TWO PLUS SIGNS on the pregnancy test turned pink, I reached for the church phone directory. Well, first I reached for the phone book (this was before internet searches were common) and looked up abortion services, the very first listing in the heavy, yellow tome. I also had to weed out the Emergency Pregnancy Centers, those anti-abortion centers with ads that read "Pregnant? Need Help?" The only help there was a fundamentalist locking me up in a room and then reciting false statistics: abortion causes breast cancer, infertility, suicide, global warming, zombie apocalypse—none of which is true. No, thank you. I knew without the slightest doubt that I wanted to end this unexpected pregnancy. I just didn't know how a person went about choosing an abortion clinic.

Today I suppose I would check out Yelp reviews, but in conservative Cleveland, abortion was something people either didn't talk about or opposed. The Catholic diocese was next to the café where I worked, and nearly every day there were protestors outside with huge photos. The barbequed baby pictures, we called them—pictures of newborn babies covered in fake blood and barbeque sauce. They were supposed to be aborted fetuses but were laughably fake. My coworkers, none of whom were particularly religious or political, joked about the pictures—but as one woman said, "I think abortion is murder. But if my teenage daughter was raped, no one would know she was pregnant but me and Planned Parenthood." A good friend had a pregnancy scare and said that while pregnancy would be a disaster, she would never do "*that*, never kill a baby." I wasn't going to call her and ask what she had heard about the various clinics, much less ask my coworkers.

The phone book listed five available clinics: two Planned Parenthoods and three independents. The listings featured a butterfly, or a pencil outline of a thin woman's body, or clouds partially covering a sun. I wondered what each one was meant to represent, what vibe the clinics were attempting. I didn't know where to go, so I grabbed my church directory and flipped through the pages.

For around six months, I'd been going to a Unitarian Universalist church in my neighborhood. It was a small congregation meeting in an old Orthodox synagogue, a funny conflation of liberal hippies in jeans and activist t-shirts, same-sex couples, and trans folks walking into an old worship space where you could still see the demarcations between the curtained women's section of the synagogue and the men's. Unitarian Universalists believe that every faith tradition holds wisdom and that reason and science are as important as religious tradition. So my UU congregation had UU-Jews and UU-Buds (Unitarian Universalist Jews and Buddhists) as well as Christians, atheists, and a huge number of agnostics. What UU congregations share is not a common theology but a common purpose—living a meaningful and ethical life. Leaving the world better than we found it. We like to say "Deeds not Creeds": don't tell me what you believe; tell me how your beliefs move you to act in the world. What we do is more important than what we believe.

I had moved on the edges of the congregation for the past half a year, falling in love with them at a rate that scared me. I had been burned by church before. I didn't trust religion or religious people. Still, I was unable to resist the pull of this congregation. From the very first Sunday, I felt a force larger than me pushing me out my door and into the sanctuary. And from the start, this quirky assortment of church folk had embraced me, inviting me to sit with them during the service, putting mugs of hot coffee into my hands at social hour, interested in the few words I shared with them.

My goal had been to hover on the edges of church life indefinitely. I didn't want any more people knowing about my screwed-up life. But without realizing it, I found myself joining a local foods potluck group, teaching Sunday School to sweet middle school kids, even sometimes singing in the choir. People asked about Drew, and I made the excuses: that he was shy, that he worked odd hours. They got the hint and stopped asking about Drew but kept engaging me. Somehow, I had become a part of this big family. Suddenly, they were my favorite people in the world, and I was happier than I had been in years. I fit somewhere. I was wanted and deeply cared for.

And I was also pregnant, damn it. The timing was awful. My marriage was disintegrating; Drew was stoned constantly. I already resented having to feed, clothe, and care for him. We were barely getting by on my meager coffee shop salary. We lived in the kind of dangerous neighborhood where kids weren't allowed to play outside at any hour. I still had panic attacks, and who knew if my depression would return?

I know that abortion stories are supposed to be full of logical reasons to end a pregnancy. Not enough money, an abusive partner, health risks. Motives listed so that a decision seems less selfish, seems like less of a choice and more of a tragedy. "I would have had that sweet little baby, but. . . ."

I had a handful of logical reasons not to want to be pregnant, but to be honest, I could have made parenthood work. I could have moved back in with my parents. Gone on low-income medical assistance. Called on aunts and uncles to babysit so I could work some job part-time. But I didn't want to be a mom. I never have. Even when playing house as a child, I wanted to be the big sister, never the mommy. I spent years caring for Drew and resenting it. I wasn't going to continue this pregnancy.

Women are taught to put other people's needs ahead of their own. That it is the natural order of things: for us to give all of our creativity and intelligence and energy, our whole selves, our whole lives, to caring for our children, spouses, and eventually aging parents. When I was little, I asked my teacher why some women didn't have children, and she said, "because they are selfish." It went against every notion of what a woman was supposed to be for me to want an abortion. I felt scalding shame over my lack of mothering instinct. Perhaps this was another facet of my mental illness? A chronic lack of a biological clock—was that in the DSM? From the moment a few days earlier when a wave of nausea made me think, *shit, am I pregnant?*, I knew I wasn't going to have a baby.

There was guilt, and plenty of shame, but no doubt. Parenthood was not in my future. I didn't have any doubts about ending the pregnancy, but I felt like I should. I felt like I should be sad, but I wasn't. I just felt relief that abortion was legal and accessible in my state. Did that make me a psychopath?

By that point, Drew and I were already in marriage counseling, although the odds looked bleaker and bleaker. I asked him if he felt guilty about my upcoming abortion. Raised Catholic, he had seen his share of barbequed baby pictures, heard sermons at mass about the sin of abortion. But he didn't feel any remorse. He said it was like I was having a root canal: it was a hassle that had to be dealt with so the condition wouldn't worsen. He didn't want to be a parent either and was relieved that, on this at least, we were in agreement. Did that make me not crazy? Or just both of us crazy?

All around us, friends and family acted like abortion was a necessary evil. Abortion was for worst-case-scenario pregnancies. But we just didn't want to have a baby. Was that a good enough reason?

Ohio's restrictive abortion laws meant I needed to hurry up and find a clinic, make an appointment, and have the procedure. I didn't know how long I had been pregnant, but after the first trimester I wouldn't be allowed to terminate my pregnancy in Ohio and would have to find the money to travel to a more woman-friendly state for the procedure. I didn't get paid time off work and wasn't sure how I was going to afford an abortion here, much less in another state. So I needed an appointment fast.

I vaguely remembered a woman at church, Martha, talking about working at an abortion clinic: about a bomb threat that had shut them down for a few hours, about the panic of patients who were terrified that the threat would bring reporters. That they might be on the news, spotted at an abortion clinic. How depressing was it that women were petrified that they would be caught having a legal medical procedure? The stigma around pregnancy termination meant that women were more worried about being seen at the clinic than about the alleged bomb.

I didn't know Martha, but we shared a church and a church family I had unwittingly fallen in love with. We were bound together by that quirky community in that old synagogue. I didn't have to know her to know that she cared about me. However, when she picked up the phone, I found myself suddenly tongue-tied. What if Martha said I didn't deserve an abortion? What if she said that my reasons weren't good enough? Maybe there was a test to pass, a test to determine if I really deserved an abortion. Would I need to prove my dire circumstances? I babbled into the phone, talking around my question, telling her I was thinking of what she had said at church about being a nurse. She asked if I was thinking of going into nursing, and I replied "No. . . ."

After a few moments of awkward silence, she said, "Oh, do you need an abortion, honey?" I said, "Yes, I need a recommendation—who has the best abortions in town?" I'm not sure what I meant by "the best," but Mary laughed and said they were all pretty good, equally safe, the same cost—but that there was a considerable shortage of abortion providers in the area and so clinics were booked up weeks in advance, if not months. She understood my worry about entering my second trimester and said she would find a time to squeeze me in at her clinic to at least see how far along I was.

A few days later, I was at the clinic getting an ultrasound. I was five weeks pregnant, an embryo smaller than a millimeter barely visible on the monitor. A tiny fleck of white on the black screen. I was tremendously relieved that I could have an abortion in my home state. It would have been nearly impossible for me to find the funds to go out of state for the procedure, and I would certainly have lost my job for missing so many days of work. But I was within the first trimester window. Exhausted from vomiting multiple times a day, charley horses, and all food tasting like metal, I scheduled my abortion for just two days later.

Abortion Day arrived humid and sunny. I was nervous; I had never had surgery or anesthesia. The nurse led me to a waiting room where, sitting in my thin hospital gown, I flipped through magazines next to another silent woman. I began to panic about the procedure—would it be painful? What if there were complications and I ended up in the hospital? Who would I have to tell then? As disastrous scenarios sped through my mind, the woman next to me began to cry.

Her hands were clasped tightly in front of her, her curly hair obscuring my view of her face. She began to sort of moan and rock back in forth. I asked her if she was okay, and she nodded yes, but her cries got louder.

"I can't believe I'm doing this. This is so messed up."

"Is someone making you? You don't have to—it's up to you."

She laughed bitterly. "Up to me. Great. Because I've done such a great job with my life so far. I have two kids. They're at school; I have to get this done with before they get out of school. I called in sick. I better not get fired."

She caught her breath, looking at me defensively. "I have to do this for my kids. I can barely feed them, keep them housed. I don't know how I'm going to buy their school supplies. This isn't a choice. I can't have a baby. We'd be on the street."

I said I was sorry, and she cried a while longer. Then, catching her breath, she said, "The thing is, I know God won't forgive me. It's not a forgivable sin. There are some rules you don't break. So I'll go to Hell. I'll go to Hell for this, ripping this baby out of me. Killing it. But I have to do it. I can't put my kids on the street."

I don't know what I replied. Her despair broke my heart. She truly believed that she was going to Hell for having an abortion, but she would choose Hell over hurting her kids. It was beautiful and terrible, this motherly sacrifice. I opened my mouth to comfort her. I wanted to talk about the God I believe in, who created abortion providers because motherhood is a sacred covenant, an agreement that not every pregnant person is in a position to make. That motherhood is a choice, and pregnancy is a question: will you continue toward parenthood? It was wonderful that she wanted to protect her two children from poverty by saying no to this pregnancy. But before I formed the words, the nurse called her into the operating room. I never saw her again.

I prayed desperately for her in the operating room, still doubting her decision. I prayed for me and for all the women and girls who have to make decisions about their bodies under enormous social and religious pressure. I prayed that we be able to hear the wisdom of our own hearts over the screaming demands of our culture that we sacrifice our own lives to care for other people. That we hear our own wisdom over the tyranny of patriarchal religions, faiths that deny the whole personhood of women, that limit their growth and freedom. In the waiting room, I was filled with gratitude for the women who worked around me in the clinic, the nurses and aides, administrators and doctors, accountants and custodians who risked social stigma and bodily harm to come to work every day so that I could be free of forced pregnancy. Our creator has gifted them with enormous bravery and graciousness.

Soon it was my turn for the operating room. I thanked God one last time for this freedom to choose or not choose motherhood and then walked inside. I laid down on the table and admitted to the nurse that I was quite nervous. She took my hand and spoke in soft, comforting tones about exactly how the operation would proceed. The doctor told me my anesthesia options, and I chose to have a local numbing agent rather than sleeping through the procedure. Sleep sounded relaxing but cost an extra $200. Soon the doctor fed a thin tube up inside my uterus. There was a loud, mechanical hum, and I felt a strong pinch in my low stomach and then cramps no worse than those during my menstrual cycle. Then the tube was coming out and the doctor said, "You are no longer pregnant!" in a celebratory way. I started to cry from relief and thanked them both profusely, and we all hugged. I said, "Thank you, thank you, thank you" to God, and then I was off to the recovery room to drink juice and eat cookies in a lounge chair.

I bled for a month afterward, every day like the heaviest day of my period. I felt 10 percent annoyed by it and 90 percent relieved that I had access to a safe, sanitary abortion. I didn't feel like I could talk to many of my friends about this life-changing procedure. I was still tender-hearted from losing my community in college when I was depressed. What if I told my friends and they rejected me? What if they said my reasons for having an abortion were not good enough?

This was the most consequential decision I had ever made, and I felt more in control of my own future than ever before. I had married due to love, sure, but also family pressure. I chose my college based on financial aid. Drew and I moved to Cleveland because he wanted to be close to his brothers. This was the first choice I had made independently, by myself and for myself alone. I felt that a rite of passage had occurred. I had come to a fork in the road and chosen a definite direction. I was proud.

I turned to my church community to celebrate. I brought Martha a homemade pie the next Sunday morning at church. When people asked why, I told some of them, the ones I trusted the most: Martha had helped me get an abortion. They hugged me. Women shared their own abortion stories and their own feelings of deep relief. We talked about God and gratitude for our freedom to choose motherhood, or not.

It is powerful to belong to a faith community that sees women as whole, holy people. We are capable of making decisions about parenthood, about pregnancy, about our future. Too many faiths seek to take away the God-given independence that strengthens women. Too many churches say that women aren't moral enough to control their own fertility, that we need laws and limits to keep us from making real choices. Motherhood is a holy covenant, not to be interfered with by men or legislation.

God didn't create women just to raise children, just to be helpmates, to serve other people. We are imbued with our own creative power. We make our own destinies. Motherhood wasn't what I wanted. I am not ashamed.

A few weeks after my abortion, when my bleeding was beginning to lessen, I had a dream. In it, I was sitting on the back steps in my parents' yard, crying, my hands covering my face. I felt a small hand shaking my shoulder and through my fingers saw a little girl, four or five, leaning in to look at me. "Mommy, mommy," she said. "It's okay, Mommy, I'm fine. I'm fine!" And then that little spirit ran away from me to spin in circles in the yard, laughing and looking at the sky.

20.

Big Sister God

THE PROBLEM WITH being married to an addict is that I stopped trusting myself. I woke to the sound of Drew filling the water bong and thought, "It isn't normal for a person to get high first thing in the morning." And in the evening, when Drew told me, full of righteous indignation, that he had been fired again, I tried to believe that it was normal to be terminated every week or so. He had lost his temper or been late, lost an important document—but it wasn't his fault, of course. I remember thinking, "How odd that a person could lose so many jobs and it be unrelated to them being high all the time."

I've heard the story, of course, of the boiled frog: if you put a frog in a pot of tepid water on the stove, he won't jump out. And if you raise the temperature slowly enough, just a few degrees at a time, he won't notice until he is boiled alive. Even with no lid on the pot, he won't jump out, because the temperature change is never extreme enough for him to be alarmed. Poor frog. I can relate. I had a happy marriage, to a sensitive, quirky, kind man. Sometimes he felt blue, or without direction. He wanted to help anyone and everyone who was suffering but didn't know how to be of use. I empathized. Now and then, he would have a few beers or a few tokes of pot to ease the harder edges of life. So did I. But then his tokes became a few a week, and then several throughout each day. Which seemed like too much to me, but Drew said he had it under control, that weed is natural, that it wasn't any different from the antidepressants I popped every morning.

And then came the day when I woke up to the water bong in use at 7 AM. I said out loud, "This isn't normal." But Drew fumed when I brought up his pot use. Drew, who had never yelled at me before, shouted about his right to get high. He said pot was no big deal, that it was my repressive parents, my Baptist upbringing skewing my mind to the conservative. Why didn't I go join Nancy Reagan's Just Say No campaign? Drew, who was never angry, would slam doors and punch the walls because his uptight wife was nagging him again about something that was no big deal. Didn't he have enough problems without my making shit up to worry about? This was my anxiety disorder making me paranoid. This had nothing to do with him. He wasn't even going to talk to me until I apologized. His friends couldn't believe the shit he had to put up with at home.

It was true that Drew's friends all smoked a lot of pot. Drew was working as a bike messenger, a job that seemed sexy and countercultural until I realized it was just schlepping briefs from one law office to another all day, back and forth across Cleveland in the bitter wind and icy snow. Poorly paid servants of the elite. His friends were messengers too, many of them selling drugs out of the biker bags that were otherwise stuffed with corporate law contracts. The messengers met up in a downtown cemetery between runs to get high, huddled close for warmth and secrecy.

Drew's friends were high all the time, so maybe it wasn't weird that he began each day with a huge hit and stayed high all day and all evening, taking a final toke on his pipe before bed. It was annoying, him being stoned constantly. I came home from my dull office job ready to cook dinner together, pull weeds together, complain about the neighbors together—the best part of being married is having someone to kvetch with—but he was glassy-eyed and dopey. Bike parts were strewn across the living room floor, and there was grease on the carpet. He took apart his bike to tune it up and then was too high to continue. Too high to have a conversation. Too high to cook or clean or buy groceries. Slowly the temperature increased in my pot of frog water, but I thought maybe it was just me being uptight. Drew said it was me being uptight. The kindest, gentlest person I knew, my husband, said I was being crazy, so I believed him.

Soon, I was the parent and Drew was the child. I handled all the household duties; he got stoned. I made money and paid bills, took care of the yard and the house and the car. Drew went to work every day, but oddly, he never brought home any money. When I asked, he got testy and shut down. I fed and clothed him, made sure he packed a healthy lunch. Made sure he went to the dentist. Bought him socks and underwear. Fielded calls from his parents, assuring them that he was fine, claiming again and again that they had just missed him, even though he was lying wide-eyed on the floor in front of me, on the grease-stained carpet. Much too stoned for a conversation.

I fielded calls from my parents, a thousand times almost asking them, "Hey, is this weird? Drew is high all the time, but he says it's no big deal—is that weird?" But I was ashamed of how bad things had gotten. I didn't want anyone to know what a trash fire our lives had become. If I confessed, certainly someone would ask why I had let it get this bad. How had I failed at emotionally supporting Drew in a way that would have kept him from being an addict? Why was I such a terrible wife? Everyone who knew Drew before he was a bike messenger knew he was whip-smart, kind, and a happy-go-lucky goofball. How had I managed to mangle him to this extreme?

I was barely holding our lives together, barely able to pay the bills. I kept the thermostat no higher than 58 degrees throughout the Cleveland winter—I couldn't afford an electric bill any higher, but any lower and the pipes would freeze. I slept in three wool sweaters and a sleeping bag under our bedspread. Drew didn't notice the cold.

I had a tight-knit group of kind friends, people who would have helped without hesitation or judgment. Friends from my Unitarian Universalist church who loved me unconditionally. Now it's hard to imagine why I didn't confide in them. There was an older woman I felt especially close to who had divorced an addict, the father of her children. She spoke about it openly and about Al-Anon—why didn't I talk with her? I just felt so ashamed. I was only twenty-four years old and my marriage was crumbling. I didn't want any witnesses to my disastrous life. There was a rich blessing of gentle souls in that congregation, but shame kept me from letting them into my reality.

I wish I had trusted them with my whole self, trusted that they would love the screwed-up real version of me as much as they loved the bubbly, happy, fake Kate that I showed them. But I didn't trust them, or anyone, really. I had lost nearly all of my college friends once word got around that I was mentally ill. Now my husband, the man who stood beside me through that loss, said his drug use was my fault. That my anxiety and my nagging were making him self-medicate. I didn't feel lovable. Once they saw me with all my faults, would they disappear too? I didn't want to risk finding out.

I was pretty mixed up about God's role in all of this. When Drew got really ticked at me, he reminded me, "You vowed for better or for worse, in sickness and in health. This is the worse. If you really believe I am addicted, you can't leave me now, because addiction is sickness. You promised God you'd stick around."

Now I can't believe I bought this bullshit. Sure, addiction is a disease, but Drew didn't want to get better. Our vows didn't say, "In sickness, including when Drew sabotages your lives over and over again, with no regard for his marriage or the well-being of his wife." Marriage vows are not an excuse to do harm. Plus, we had promised to honor and love each other, and I was feeling neither of those. But at the time, my self-esteem was gutted by my depression, anxiety, and abandonment by my college friends. God and I were just getting reacquainted and I was starting to pray again. I sat in church and begged God to make Drew stop smoking pot. I bargained: "Anything you want, God, I'll do anything. You name it. You make Drew stop smoking and I'll do anything." Then I went to coffee hour and pretended that my life was just fine. I smiled and laughed and refused to let my church family see my whole self.

One Sunday afternoon I loaded the laundry into our shitty car and took it to the shitty laundromat, where there was always a cop stationed outside the door, sometimes two. Drew had previously handled the laundry because of the sketchiness of this establishment, where I was offered drugs in exchange for sex acts, cash, or laundry detergent. But that was the old Drew. Now he was too stoned to drive, and when I asked him about the mountains of laundry piling up, he snapped about me nagging. So, ignoring the other clientele, I began emptying Drew's corduroy trousers into a jumbo washer. In the pockets were a plastic baggie of weed, a small purple glass pipe, and a pretty wooden box I had never seen, packed with weed. In his jeans I discovered rolling papers and a cheap plastic lighter with neon pink hearts. I glanced up at the cops talking to each other by the door and then down at my hands, full of illegal drugs and drug paraphernalia. This was before pot was decriminalized. I was holding enough evidence to get me a few weeks in jail. Definitely an arrest that would end my employment, the only job bringing money into our household.

This was my lightning-bolt moment. God, in her no-nonsense, feisty-big-sister voice, said, "Seriously, are you going to keep enabling this shit? Do you think I created you to put up with this garbage?" God yanked me out of my stupor. The truth she unveiled was painful. Was I really hiding my husband's drugs from the police because he was too stoned to clean out his pockets? When had this become our lives? I wrapped the pot, the wooden box, the pink lighter, and the purple pipe in Drew's favorite t-shirt. Then, when the police were looking the other direction, I dumped it all in the jumbo trash can in the corner.

When I got home, Drew and I had a big fight. Reality had solidified at the laundromat. Goddess had spoken. This couldn't be normal. I could have gotten arrested. When did he become so addicted that every pair of pants had pot in the pockets? Drew said I was crazy, of course. He said it was my anxiety disorder making me freak out, that his behavior was normal. I cried. I never thought he would use my mental illness against me. He said it was my fault he smoked all the time because taking care of me made him so stressed out. I cried some more. He said I was overreacting, that pot was no big deal, but I told him the time for that bullshit argument had passed. I cried like there was no bottom to my grief, so hysterically that Drew worried the neighbors would hear me wailing like a banshee.

My grief had finally been uncorked and there was no stopping the flow of tears and snot flowing from my face. I fell on the floor and curled into a ball, seeking comfort in the fetal position. I thrashed out at Drew's hand on my back. How dare he? How dare he try to calm me when he had made me doubt my own sanity for months? Seasons had passed that he spent stoned and convincing me I was overreacting. That my anxiety disorder was the problem. Grief and rage tossed me back and forth while I wailed. I couldn't breathe. I was lost in the feelings I had been denying for over a year. I was above my body, looking down at a soul writhing in pain. A damned soul that somehow had my own face.

Drew was overwhelmed. He stepped outside into the winter night, and the frigid wind blowing in through the door brought me to my senses. I rose and, in a weary voice that brooked no argument, informed him that he would see his doctor to talk about addiction and that we were going to start marriage counseling. He didn't reply. I went upstairs, falling immediately into a deep and dreamless quicksand of sleep.

In the morning it was hard to free myself from slumber. Reality was an unappealing spotlight focused on the wreckage of our life together. I couldn't look away. Denial was now inconveniently unavailable. I would stay trapped no longer.

That evening I told Drew that I had made him a doctor's appointment, and he said he didn't want to go. I lifted my eyebrows and looked at the place on the floor where I had become a banshee, and he said he would go to the doctor but not to marriage counseling. So I told him everything: that I was desperately lonely when he was near me because he was too stoned to really be with me. That I didn't want to be his parent. That I was tired of keeping our household, and his whole life, running while he stared into space every day. That I was furious that I was paying all the bills and had no idea where his money was going. He tried to interrupt, to argue that no one had asked me to be his mother, to pay the bills—but I was too tired to argue and just plowed through his words with my own.

I told him it wasn't normal to be stoned all day every day and, that yes, I knew his friends were stoned all the time, but I didn't want to live like them. I frankly didn't like them, these grubby men who frequently sprawled out on our living room floor, endlessly discussing the superiority of fixed-gear bicycles. They disparaged the office workers they saw rushing around downtown, who worked for the man and were stuck commuting by car. "Cars are coffins!" they would shout at the suit-clad public, weaving their bikes through jammed intersections, running red lights, riding against traffic. These cool-obsessed bike messengers, grown men who had fathered children they didn't see or pay to support, who were proud they weren't selling out to convention. They were toddler-like in their grasping of pleasure and rejection of responsibility. I had no interest in whether they smoked pot all day because I had no affection or even respect for them. Their normal could no longer be our normal.

Then Drew came to the big "Or what?" I had insulted Drew's friends, admitting that I was disappointed that he chose to spend time with them. I wanted him to pay bills, to clean and cook, to be sober enough to have conversations. To act like a husband and not like a child. I wanted him to talk to his doctor about his addiction to marijuana, and I wanted marriage counseling because our relationship was screwed up to the point of being nearly unfixable. Drew looked at me with his sea-glass-green eyes and said, "Or what?"

Or what. Or what. I knew what I would do if Drew didn't change, but I was afraid to say it. We had never had a big enough fight to use the D-word, never had a rough enough spell to invoke the legal ending of our marriage. I thought we were unbreakable, and I knew Drew did as well.

Mentioning divorce felt like letting an evil spirit into our sanctuary, like once the word was said it would become inevitable. Divorce. If I said it, it would happen.

"If things don't change, I am leaving." Close enough to saying the D-word. Drew stormed out of the house.

The next week, Drew and I sat inside a crystal-filled room in a chi-chi suburb of Cleveland. The marriage counselor saw her clients in an office at the front of her house, a huge Tudor with prissy landscaping that clashed with the hippie/new age décor inside. She was a short woman in a silky purple muumuu and reading glasses with purple rhinestones on the frames, which clacked pleasingly against the purple crystal earrings dangling from her lobes. She looked like a very kind witch. I could tell Drew hated her on sight, but that felt inevitable.

The counselor came highly recommended by the very few people that Drew allowed me to ask for recommendations, since he didn't want people to know that we were having problems. Her fee was a month's worth of groceries, but I happily forked it over in the hopes that her witchy magic would fix us. For the first ten minutes she asked us a million rapid-fire questions: where we were from, if our parents were married, what we did for a living. It lulled us into answering her questions without hesitation, so we were primed when she dove into the hard stuff: Why were we seeking counseling? I said Drew's drug problem. Drew said my anxiety over his casual drug use and need to control everything. Had one of us had an affair? Nope, I said, with Drew overlapping, "No, we managed to fuck up our marriage without help from outsiders." Was one of us unhappy about being in counseling? she asked, with a pointed look at Drew. "Wow, you're good at this," replied Drew sarcastically. "Are we fixed now?"

We filled our fifty-minute session with the polite, furious conversation of good Midwesterners who were taught not to yell but really want to. As the timer chimed, our good witch/therapist flipped closed her notebook and gave us each thirty seconds of intense, uncomfortable eye contact. Then she sighed and said, "You love each other. You communicate well. There isn't anything wrong with your relationship—" (Drew started to rise) "—but Drew" (significant pause and eye contact), "you are addicted to pot and need to quit. It's going to wreck your life. Kate can help you, but you have to want to quit. I can keep seeing you together, but it won't help. The problem isn't you two, it's the drug use."

It was very difficult for me to restrain my jubilation at this news. I wanted to pump my arms and cheer: it isn't us! It's the drugs! Easy-peasy fix—he would quit, we would heal, get old together, happily ever after, matching rocking chairs on the porch as we whiled away our golden years. Awesome!

Drew said, "This is bullshit, and you are crazy. I'm leaving." And Midwest politeness be damned, he actually left.

And my happy fantasy of us holding hands on the porch in our dotage disappeared.

So began our tour of Greater Cleveland–area marriage therapists. I would track down a recommended therapist, fork over a month's worth of grocery money for the session, and the counselor would conclude that our relationship wasn't the problem, drugs were the problem. Drew would get angry and leave. And I would find another therapist. Because denial ain't just a river in Egypt.

I loved Drew deeply, and our early years together had been incredibly sweet, so I kept trying to believe that one of the therapists would have the magic words to convince him he needed help. If we found the right therapist, someone he liked and related to, he would hear the truth and believe it. On more clear-headed days I knew that no individual therapist could sway him but still thought that maybe the quantity of therapists all saying the same thing would convince him. He needed more evidence than his lost jobs, his angry wife, the disappearance of his non-pothead friends. . . . But in the meantime, we wasted fistfuls of money seeing counselors he didn't believe.

My motives were not entirely pure. I truly wanted to spend the rest of my life at Drew's side. I believed in him. That his kindness and intelligence would somehow heal a bit of the world that was breaking his heart. I loved him and I really, really liked him too—when he wasn't stoned, he was funny and sharp and creative. He had unique ideas and a big heart. It felt good to be near him. I missed the Drew that I fell in love with. I needed to believe that he would return.

But frankly, I also didn't know how I could cope without him. From the outside, I was very healthy: no anxiety attacks, depression managed with pharmaceuticals and lots of jogging and yoga. I was tightly held in a loving church community; I had just gotten a big promotion at work. But inside, my utter breakdown of three years before hovered just out of sight. It felt so nearby, like I could fall apart at any moment. That I could wake up one day and want to die, that the crushing, unrelenting pain of existence with depression could swoop in and carry me away. And how could I manage that pain without Drew?

Losing nearly all of my friends in college left me untrusting of friendships in general. Drew stayed with me when I was hospitalized, all three times. He visited me in three different lock-down psych wards. He was patted down by security before sitting with me as I wept hysterically for our entire visit. He borrowed cars from friends and drove three hours across snowy Ohio to see me for two hours. His girlfriend in a hospital gown, with the shakes and toxic breath from the medications. I would wail "I want to die" while in his arms, and he quietly cried, but he didn't leave. He didn't break up with me. Even when I begged him to, so sure was I that I was a burden—the side effect of depression that made me believe everyone would be better off without me. He assured me that I would get better. He repeated it like a mantra, and sometimes I even believed him. He said he loved me no matter what. Even if I was like this forever, he was sticking around. Often, his words gave me my only peace.

When my best friends kicked me out of our shared house, when my closest friends wouldn't even make eye contact as I pleaded for a second chance, Drew carried my mattress and clothes and books across campus to his house and installed me there. He told his roommates not to be weird around me and made me macaroni and cheese for dinner. He held me every night as I cried myself to sleep. He learned about meditation so he could teach me to do it. He loved me so much that I slowly began to love myself again.

Perhaps surprisingly, I didn't feel like I owed it to Drew to stay in our marriage. Yes, I wanted to honor our wedding vows, the promises we made to each other. But I hadn't married him to pay back some sort of balance he had accrued with his kindness when I was ill. He was good to me during my hardest period because he is a deeply caring and generous person, not because he wanted me to owe him or to lock me into an obligatory relationship. But I did fear deeply, in the reptilian center of my brain, that if he and I parted and then I got depressed again, no one but my biological family would ever accept me again. No one would love me who wasn't required to by blood ties. How could I trust my friends when friends had betrayed me before? How could I leave the only nonbiological relative who loved me unconditionally?

At the same time, being so terribly depressed in my recent past showed me the preciousness of regular life. I worried I could fall into a depression again at any time. Mentally healthy life was not to be taken for granted; it could vanish with a change in brain chemistry. This lonely life with Drew wasn't a good use of healthy time. I had worked determinedly to recover. A team of people had struggled to get me well. Was this how I was going to spend the life that was so hard earned?

My savings account dwindled until we didn't have the funds to see another private-practice therapist. Catholic Charities set us up with a young woman just out of school, earning her mental health credentials and willing to see us for a pittance. Drew and I went through our regular spiel, well rehearsed by this time: the history of our relationship, what we each thought the problem was. But this novice therapist came to a new conclusion. She said okay, Kate says too much weed, Drew says it's not too much weed. Wife says addict, husband says just recreational use. You two aren't going to come to a conclusion on the too much/not too much debate. So, what is it you each want?

Drew said that he wanted me to chill out about his drug use and quit worrying so much. I said I wanted him to quit smoking pot. Same old stalemate. It seemed that I had wasted another hour of my life, but fortunately not the standard $120, on this session. But then she said, "So what happens if he doesn't quit, Kate?" After a long pause, I repeated the ultimatum I had gravely stated months before: if he doesn't quit, I'm leaving.

"When?" she asked. I just looked at her. "When? What is the time frame? If he doesn't quit by x date, then you will leave. Let's be as specific as possible. Drew doesn't think he is an addict, so he needs to know what is at stake if he doesn't change. When will you leave?"

"Four months." It just popped out. It was exactly four months until my birthday. "If the pot isn't out of our lives in four months, I'm leaving. You can taper off of it until then, but on my birthday it is completely gone."

I felt an enormous relief at setting a date. I was sure Drew would stop now that he knew I would leave. Now that a date loomed, I felt at peace. Drew rolled his eyes and said that in four months I would be over worrying about this and onto some other pointless concern, but I could tell that he was apprehensive. The crease between his eyes tensed as he contemplated the nearness of the deadline. Still, I knew he would quit. Look how much we had overcome in our relationship! He had loved me through a mental breakdown. The man was clearly crazy about me. He would quit, and we would heal.

We talked about recovery, AA meetings, meds his doctor could prescribe. But Drew said he didn't need any of it, he wasn't addicted, he could just stop. But he still didn't want to stop. So the counselor circled back: "Okay, you aren't addicted. But if you don't stop, Kate is leaving. Is it worth stopping to stay married?"

"Sure, but I shouldn't have to stop."

"But if you don't stop, Kate is leaving. So, will you stop?"

"This is bullshit, I'm not addicted."

'That's fine, you don't have to be addicted—but will you stop?"

"I shouldn't have to stop. I'm not addicted, she worries too much."

"I hear you saying that, but Kate is leaving if you don't stop smoking pot. So will you stop?"

The therapist and Drew circled around like this through several sessions. I just watched, marveling at her tenacity. Finally, about two months before the deadline, Drew agreed to taper down his pot use so that he would be off of it by my birthday.

It didn't work, this deadline. The week after my birthday I moved in with friends from church, Lala and Diane, a nice couple with an extra bedroom. I repaid them by crying loudly at all hours and offering no rent. I thought that if I moved out, Drew would be so shocked at my absence, so sad missing me, that he would quit smoking weed and we could get better. But while he professed to missing me, he didn't quit, and decided he didn't want to quit. On a cold January day, ice making the windows look like diamonds, we met in the chilly courthouse in downtown Cleveland and got a divorce. I cried so hard I vomited. He didn't know what to say.

Sadly, that was the last time I saw Drew. I hoped we would eventually be friends, but he was awfully angry at me for going through with the divorce. I don't think he believed I would do it. I like to imagine that if we lived in the same city we would hang out, that his wife and family would hang out with me and Jay, my current husband. Perhaps it is a good thing that we live on opposite sides of the country now so I can keep that fantasy alive. I am not angry anymore.

21.

Starting Single

WHEN I WAS FOUR OR FIVE, I loved to spin around in circles until I got so dizzy that I fell down. Then I would lie on the ground, laughing, as the world seemingly spun above me. That is the feeling that I had after I got divorced, minus the laughing. The world spun and I had no balance, lying on the ground trying to make sense of a new reality.

I took up jogging in the last months of my marriage to manage the panic attacks that came in crashing waves whenever I let myself realize that my marriage was ending. I ran five miles a day trying to escape my anxiety, but often I started crying as soon as I stopped moving. One day, shortly after moving in with Lala and Diane, I went on a long run and as soon as I got home, I collapsed in a heap of tears on the porch. I thought I was the only one home, but Lala came outside and nudged me with her foot to see what was going on. I looked up at her and said, "Drew used to make me smoothies after I ran. Now who is going to do it?"

Lala, normally very sympathetic, said, "You can make your own damn smoothies. I'll dig out the blender," and headed to the basement. This was how post-divorce life seemed to work: I would realize that I was on my own in making a decision or doing something simple like mixing fruit and juice in a blender. I would cry for a while as it hit me, again, that Drew was gone, and then get on with figuring out how to do it on my own. Life called me forward with its practical needs. I didn't know how to cook, since Drew had liked making dinner, but I learned. I didn't know what to do when the oil light came on in my car, but it turns out I could pay someone to change my oil. As the weeks passed I realized that, after I cried, I could figure out most problems.

The biggest question was what I was going to do with my life. In church on the Sunday after my divorce, I heard the Mary Oliver poem "Wild Geese" that ends, "What will you do with your one wild and precious life?" Before I chose to have an abortion, I felt like life was something that happened to me and that I reacted to. But now I was beginning to feel like I could be the catalyst. My congregation had built me up with their love and I was feeling more confident than at any time since the Big Depression. Sure, I had panic attacks and crying jags, but they were because of getting divorced. My heart was slowly healing. I felt powerful in a new way.

Who did I want to be? When I was around nine, I started thinking about being a minister. The women I admired the most were my ministers, and it felt like their job was to love the congregation and help us grow spiritually and morally. That seemed like a pretty neat job. Then I had the Big Depression and got mad at God and religion and anything that seemed spiritual. But faith and I had reconciled. I loved being a Unitarian Universalist and exploring religion from every possible angle. I loved that our worship services incorporated Carl Sagan and Bikini Kill lyrics and the Buddha. Could I be a UU minister?

It wasn't a decision I wanted to rush. After all, I was broke and newly single and making minimum wage. So I decided my first step toward whatever the future held was to get a better-paying job and pay off my student loans. Then I would have more flexibility if I wanted to go to graduate school. Meanwhile, I would go to church and meditate and try to listen for the possibilities my life could hold.

I got a terribly dull but well-paying job in a corporate office downtown. It was like being thrust into the comic strip *Dilbert*: inept bosses and angry underlings, wars over staplers and whose turn it was to make coffee. I didn't care; it was temporary. I was on a spiritual quest, and this was just paying the bills. I got a promotion and while in a restroom stall heard a coworker say it was because I was a "ball-buster," which made me laugh. I was just there to pay off my student loans.

Meanwhile, I had been with my church a few years and was singing in the choir, teaching Sunday school, and leading a young adult group. I was surprised but flattered when I was asked to join the Board of Trustees, which in my childhood congregation was a really big honor. I accepted the position and learned everything I could about church board leadership and Unitarian Universalism so I would be prepared. Then I learned that being on the board wasn't a big deal in this congregation and that they had asked many people, all of whom said no, before they asked me—but no matter. I loved my scrappy little congregation and was going to give it my all.

It was a joyful way to serve the community and a wonderful escape from the corporate mindset I used during the day. At work, it was all about money: saving money, making money, reducing overhead, profit margins. It was easy to forget that money wasn't the only lens through which to see value. Unitarian Universalists, on the other hand, are inspired by Seven Principles, seven life-guiding tenets for making decisions.

First Principle: The inherent worth and dignity of every person;

Second Principle: Justice, equity, and compassion in human relations;

Third Principle: Acceptance of one another and encouragement to spiritual growth in our congregations;

Fourth Principle: A free and responsible search for truth and meaning;

Fifth Principle: The right of conscience and the use of the democratic process within our congregations and in society at large;

Sixth Principle: The goal of world community with peace, liberty, and justice for all;

Seventh Principle: Respect for the interdependent web of all existence of which we are a part.

We used these tenets in coming to verdicts on the Board. Was our decision just? Was it compassionate? Would it encourage spiritual growth and acceptance of one another? Did it honor every person's inherent worth and dignity while respecting the web of all existence?

Was it cheesy? Hell yes. But for an idealist turned cynic who was trying to figure out what really mattered, it was life changing. It was useful idealism. It was so much better than making choices based on how much cash it would raise for shareholders. I joined the Board because I loved my congregation and wanted to serve—and it was a huge ego boost to be asked. But on the Board, I learned a whole new way of structuring my decision making.

While on the Board I thought about a lot of different careers—librarian, speech pathologist, drama teacher, social worker. All of those jobs would have been fine choices, fulfilling roles that probably would have made me happy. But when I thought about what I would do with my time if I found out I had six months to live, it would be to spread Unitarian Universalism. And when I thought about what I would do if I won a million dollars, it would be to spread Unitarian Universalism. I have no doubt that humanity would be happier, fairer, and more ecologically friendly if there were more UUs. When I reached for a book, it was on theology, and when I met a friend for coffee, we talked about justice and equality. It was time to apply for seminary.

22.

Once Burned, Twice Shy

JUST BEFORE DREW AND I got divorced, I called his mom to say goodbye. She is a wild, creative, kind, intellectual whirlwind of a woman, a computer programmer and fiber artist who worked on the first incarnations of the internet while weaving baskets out of tree bark and raising three hippie boys who are peace-loving feminists. She is deeply religious and practices her faith in the Catholic tradition in which she was brought up, although she disagrees with every other thing her priest says. I knew we could and would talk again after the divorce, but I also knew that our relationship would change. She always called me "her first girl" since she had three sons and then finally a daughter-in-law. I felt unconditional love for her, inspired by her unconditional love for me. But I was leaving her son, and he was hurt and very angry. I was choosing to leave her family. I loved them, and the grief was a heavy blanket over my head. It was time to say goodbye to being her first girl.

We talked, we cried, we laughed a little and then cried a lot more. And then she told me she hoped I would fall in love again soon. I laughed. "I am never, ever falling in love again." And she got very quiet. "No, Kate, no. You are good at being in love. You were good at being married. Don't let this stop you."

Then I was crying harder than I thought possible. "But it's over. I did everything I could, everything I could think of. I read all the books and went to all the therapists. I was patient and kind and mean and bossy. Nothing worked. And it hurts *so much*. I could never survive this kind of pain again."

I meant it at the time. The end of my marriage was so painful that many times I was shocked that the emotional pain couldn't kill me. How could I still be grocery shopping, going to work, making dinner (I mean, dinner was usually cereal, but still), moving in the world when I felt like a giant open wound being scraped with sandpaper? I was done with love. I had friends I adored, a terrific family. I didn't need to fall in love and potentially go through this agony again.

"Kate, listen to me." This was the most serious I had ever heard her sound, the most resolute. "Listen—love is going to come to you again. Just be open to it. You can't live your life afraid."

Ha! Shows how much she knows, I thought. I spent lots of my life afraid. That's what life is like with an anxiety disorder. But through my haze of grief, I heard her.

Dating was still the last thing I wanted to do. I was enveloped in the tender care of Lala and Diane, who were devoted to getting me through my sadness one bowl of ice cream and *Northern Exposure* rerun at a time. They were patient with my constant crying and dragged me out for walks when I spent too long inside in my dark room. I wasn't leaving them until it was time for seminary, and that was only if I couldn't find a way to get them to move with me.

Almost a year after my conversation with my ex–mother-in-law, when I was starting to feel happy and confident again, Lala and Diane threw a party. They had legendary parties. Being genuinely curious about every person they met, and uninterested in the sorts of social boundaries that usually keep classes and races apart, they had fascinating friends. Diane and Lala would put out platters of food, and everyone would bring oodles of wine and spread out across the porch and living room talking and dancing long into the night.

Jay came to the party that night. Jay and I had been friends for a few years, distant friends since he lived an hour away and preferred staying home and making art to socializing. We met at Summer Institute, an all-ages Unitarian Universalist summer camp that gathered people from several states, and at the time people teased Jay about being the only single straight guy at camp. Jay was teaching a mosaic class that a friend of mine was in, so we ended up eating several meals together, and I thought he was funny in a super-wholesome way. I decided to set him up with a single friend who was also an artist.

The first setup didn't work; Serena thought he was too quiet. That was true: Jay is very quiet. I set him up with Rose, but she said he was too unfocused, didn't have any ambition. Also true, but I saw that as his not being materialistic. Then Jay said he would find his own girlfriends and to please stop setting him up. We hadn't really spent much time together since them.

When Jay arrived at the party, I was passing out a big platter of tiny, colorful ice cream sandwiches. I didn't see him approach, but when he was about two feet away, I turned around and looked him right in the eyes and felt electricity jolt down my legs and back up through my head. I couldn't form words—what the hell was going on with me?—so I just gave him a half smile and moved away. But wherever I moved, I could feel this electricity zinging between us, like a cord of heat tying us together. With my back to him, I felt him move around the room, getting a drink, talking to various friends. I felt so self-conscious, like he was taking in my every move, but when I turned around, he wasn't even looking my direction.

I considered slipping off to change clothes. I was in baggy shorts and a t-shirt. I hadn't thought about dating in a year, so I didn't dress to impress anyone, ever. I had sneakers on, my legs were hairy, and suddenly I cared what I looked like. Suddenly I wanted to look attractive. What the hell was going on?

It got late and the party wound down. Soon it was just Lala, Diane, Jay, and me. Lala said she was taking the dog for a walk, and we all decided to go along. As we walked, Diane and Jay ended up about ten feet in front of Lala and me. I still felt the electric zing going between us. I asked Lala if Jay was dating anyone. She said not that she knew of and then looked thoughtful. "Hmm. Yeah, I can see you two together."

I rolled my eyes and said it wasn't like that, and Lala was kind enough to pretend to believe me. But the next day I called Jay to see if he wanted to go to a movie, and he said yes.

There were many bumps on the way to our falling in love. I was still terrified of getting hurt, so we took the relationship at a glacial pace. We dated for four years before we lived together. Still, he moved to Boston to be near me during seminary. He was endlessly supportive of my desire to be a UU minister, since Unitarian Universalism is a big part of his life. In 2015, after Marriage Equality was finally made law, we got married. I am glad every day that I married him and that we get to travel this life together.

23.

Fasten Your
Theological Seatbelt

IT WAS DAY ONE of Hebrew Bible, a required class that most students take in their first semester of seminary. I was in the front row, with my pens laid out neatly and a fresh notebook open. The class was full of both new friends I had met in my four days on campus and strangers, all of us looking around nervously and wondering if we were really smart enough for graduate school.

I attended Andover Newton Theological School in suburban Boston, Massachusetts. Andover Newton is a multifaith seminary, which just meant that Unitarian Universalists shared classes with Christians from many denominations, mostly the mainline liberal ones. A rabbinical school was next door, and we shared social events with them. Andover Newton is historically American Baptist, and most of the faculty are Christians who are used to teaching Christians, but recently the school had begun recruiting UUs.

There are two UU seminaries, Starr King in Berkeley, California, and Meadville Lombard in Chicago, Illinois. I had assumed I would attend one of those schools, but neither could offer me any scholarships, and when I looked at Craigslist to see how much apartments in Berkeley cost, I thought there was an error in the algorithm and an extra zero had been added to each price. While initially I was disappointed not to attend a UU school—they are both academically rigorous and well respected—I liked the feel of Andover Newton. It was on a big, wooded hill and felt separated from the real world. The campus was all red-brick buildings around a leafy green quad, with white Adirondack chairs full of students debating or dozing in the sun. At the top of the quad was the chapel, a modern glass and steel structure in the shape of a traditional New England church. It was the definition of charming.

As Hebrew Bible class began, I learned first that the Hebrew Bible is what we used to call the Old Testament, changed because "Old Testament" infers that there is a new, better testament, and that is disrespectful of the Jewish tradition. Also, the Hebrew Bible text was in Hebrew and is the primary text for Jews. Calling it the Hebrew Bible is more factually correct and a good reminder about how the whole Christianity thing sprang up (from Jesus, a Jew). I scribbled all that into my notebook, feeling relieved that I was keeping up, but the professor was just getting started.

Did you know that there are at least four creation stories in Genesis? Neither did I. Did you know that there are references to sea monsters and to other gods? Again, neither did I. But soon we were diving into the two most popular creation stories, which I call "And it was good" (God separates the sky from the water, light from dark, etc., and it was good) and "Adam and Eve" (God makes Adam from Eve's rib because Adam is lonely). A hand was raised. "Professor, how do these stories work together? They seem mutually exclusive—how are they both true?"

This question caused the professor to stop and peer over his small wire-rimmed glasses at us. He sighed deeply and said, "They don't fit together. And they aren't both true, not in a factual way. They are both stories about how people imagined the world started. God didn't write the Bible, people did. And [an even bigger sigh] seminary is going to be hard on those of you who have a Sunday School faith. There is nothing wrong with you, but if you haven't thought about the Bible critically before, fasten your seatbelt because here comes a bumpy ride."

He wasn't kidding. Turns out a lot of kind, smart people come to seminary with nothing but Sunday School faith. And so when they learn about the conflicting creation stories, about the sea monsters in the Bible, the dragons, about how originally the book of John ended with Christ not being resurrected but lying dead in a tomb . . . they flip out. In class. Some students put their heads on their desks and cry; some just leave the classroom, pack up their room, and leave campus for good. Some try to stick out the semester and then go. Wrestling with faith is never easy, but it is harder when you find out how flimsy your belief is when you are in the middle of a class that is supposed to lead to your being a minister.

It turns out that seminaries have a high dropout rate. I hope the students who left continued to explore faith and God. I know what it is like to be bitter about religion; I don't recommend it. For those of us who stayed, the theological difficulties continued. One day in Hebrew Bible class our professor mentioned an ancient Assyrian text that had a flood story similar to that of Noah and the Ark. I asked, "When do we study the ancient Assyrian religion? I want to know more about that."

He gave me his now familiar look over his small wireframe glasses and sighed. "Let me guess: you are a Unitarian Universalist?" I nodded yes, and he began to sing,

"Come home, coooommeee homeeee to Je-e-sus."

I rolled my eyes and he said, "This is a Christian seminary. It has always been a Christian seminary. That isn't changing just because you UUs are here. You want to learn about Assyrians, go to an Assyrian seminary."

"But we are studying ancient Jewish texts in this class. Shouldn't we do that at a rabbinical school?" I countered. The professor threw a marker at me, laughed, and got back to the lesson. But it wasn't the first time I encountered bias against UU students.

Some of my classmates thought that since we are a non-creedal religion, we don't believe anything. In creedal religions, a person has to agree to a list of religious beliefs in order to be a part of a congregation. Think of the Apostles' Creed: agreeing to that means agreeing that you believe a set of theological principles, like that there is one God, that Jesus is the son of that God, and that Jesus was crucified and resurrected. The idea is that everyone in that church, and in the denomination, agree that a list of statements is correct. On Sundays they get together to reaffirm those beliefs and their central place in believers' lives. The clergyperson's goal is to convince people to believe these central tenets so they can live a morally correct life and get into heaven. Church as fire insurance, I joke.

In UU churches we don't ask people to agree to a set of beliefs in order to belong to a congregation. We meet each week to consider different ideas, to explore if they are true for us personally. We ask church members to agree that they will explore religious belief in a way that is respectful to people who believe differently than they do. We believe that all religions have aspects of truth; that faith, science, and reason are all good ways to discover life's meaning. Service and justice making are how we practice our faith. Trying to make the world better for every creature is the goal of our spiritual life. We UUs don't share a belief about what happens when we die, but we agree that life is hellish for plenty of people here on earth, and we want to remedy that.

In seminary my religious beliefs evolved and grew, and so did my respect for my Christian classmates. I am continually inspired by liberal Christians' devotion to trying to live like Jesus—giving to the poor, making peace, living simply with few possessions. Their faith inspires them, and me, to live in the model of that great Jewish prophet. But I know that relegating my spiritual search to one faith, to any one faith, would not be satisfying to me. After all, the Bible wasn't written by God—no religious ideas come from the Source. It's all just what different people, at different times in history, in different parts of the world, theorized about the great mystery that is God. All of those ideas, plus science, plus my own explorations of the world, create in me a sense of boundless wonder and love for humanity. What could be holier than that?

24.

Like in Washington?

I SPENT FOUR GLORIOUS YEARS in seminary and completing a ministry internship. It was a difficult, joyful, precious time, perhaps the best four years of my life so far. But as graduation loomed large, I began the formal search process of looking for a UU congregation to serve. The search system is a lot like online dating—ministers put up a short profile of information about their experience and theology. Congregations put up a brief outline detailing what is important to them and what they are looking for in a minister. Then if the minister likes the congregation, and the congregation likes the minister, a more detailed packet of information is exchanged—a hundred pages or so of sample sermons and statements of belief from the ministers, church financial statements, and Board minutes from the congregations. It all takes about five months and culminates in the minister's spending a week with the congregation, preaching twice and meeting all the committees and various affinity groups. Then the whole congregation votes. If they vote yes, the new ministry begins in a few months. If they vote no, the whole process starts again.

It is quite stressful. All through seminary we heard about how difficult it would be to find a ministry position, how there were twice as many ministers as jobs for ministers, how new ministers have to serve congregations in places where other people don't want to move. Jay was at that time in graduate school for mental health counseling, preparing to be the therapist he is today. So that he could finish his master's degree, we only looked at congregations in places where there was a graduate program in psychology. It's a popular field so that didn't limit the field much, fortunately. I posted my profile to the search site, and we started looking at the congregations that needed ministers. We were determined not to be choosy, lest I not get a job.

I checked that I was interested in about eighteen different congregations in places all over the United States. Some were associate or assistant positions, working with a senior minister. Many were in small towns in the Midwest where the cost of living would be nice and low, but Jay might have a hard time finding a job when he got out of school. Only one was in a big city, and it seemed like a long shot at best. A congregation in Shoreline, Washington, just outside the city of Seattle. The search committee posted a picture on the search site of a huge white mountain surrounded by pine trees, overlooking a large city on a long harbor. Seattle. There was no way they were going to pick a brand new minister with no experience. But why not apply? When I asked Jay what he thought about living in Seattle, he said, "In Washington? No way." It was too good to be a real option. I confirmed that I meant Seattle, Washington, and Jay, who rarely swears, said "Hell yes."

Eleven congregations requested my search packet, which was a good sign. But only seven requested a phone interview, which was a bad sign. With other friends who were in search, I worried over every little thing that a search committee said. It was just like dating. "What do you think they meant when they said they lean humanist but are open? Why did they ask so many questions about Jay? Did it seem like there were a lot of long silences during the interview? Did I make too many jokes?"

Finally, the second-to-last stage arrived: in-person interviews. Five search committees asked me to come interview with them. In retrospect, I should have narrowed it down to three, but I was unsure of what I wanted and terrified I wouldn't get anything, so I went on so many interviews that I kept mixing up the details of different congregations. It was embarrassing. But Shoreline, Washington, was my favorite congregation for a simple reason: they admitted that they had made mistakes. When I asked about a dip in attendance I saw in their records or a budget shortfall, their search committee would say, "Yes, we tried this new thing, and it didn't work, and we learned a lot." It felt like a place where it would be safe to be an inexperienced new minister.

I knew I was going to make errors; I made piles and piles of them in my internship. I said something that hurt someone's feelings or forgot to go to a meeting. One night we had a Passover supper and I grabbed a big jug of grape juice, labeled only in Hebrew, and poured little cups for the kids. One of the kids took a sip and said it tasted weird—it was red wine. I wanted a congregation where I could be wrong and not get fired.

Finally it was Call Day, the day when search committees could offer a position to the minister of their choice. I cried when Shoreline UU called and asked me to be their minister. It felt like the satisfaction of sliding a final puzzle piece into place. I called Jay the second he was out of class to tell him we were moving to Seattle. "Yes!" he yelled. "Hell yes!"

25.

The Dalai Lama Says I'm Okay. My Niece Disagrees.

THREE YEARS AGO, I got to officiate the marriage of my brilliant, smart-ass brother to a brilliant, smart-ass woman. Now they have this fantastic daughter, the smartest, coolest, sweetest infant who has ever lived. I don't have kids, and this is my brother's first, so everyone in my family adores her like she is the second coming of Christ (which—who knows? The world could do worse).

A few months ago, I was holding my niece with one arm and balancing a cup of lukewarm coffee in my other hand. I looked away for just a second—I feel like all baby stories start this way—I looked away for just one second and she stuck her little pink fist right into my coffee cup. She yanked it back out and gave me the dirtiest look I have ever received. How DARE you hold tepid coffee near me! She took a really long, deep breath—never a good sign, I've learned— and then let out an even longer wail. I was bouncing her and singing a comforting little song and frantically looking for a dish towel when she jammed her other little pink fist into the mug. Now she was waving her tiny hands in pro- test and looking at me with such disgust, such disappoint- ment, like, "What the hell is the matter with you? And why would my parents ever leave me with such an idiot?"

She wasn't burned, just mad at being wet, I suppose. Who knows? But I couldn't help but laugh—Lovebug, why did you stick your other hand in? Did you think it would be different the second time? Oh, you little goofball. That was a silly thing to do.

When children do silly things, it is so forgivable. How can you be mad at someone who genuinely doesn't know that they shouldn't stick their fists in a coffee cup? How can you be mad at the ridiculousness of human nature—that we make the same mistakes over and over, even when we are babies? Even when we should know better.

It is so easy to see the Buddha-nature in children. Do you know that word, *Buddha-nature*? The direct translation varies based on who you ask; Buddhist ideas are translated differently in different parts of the world. But, at its essence, it means the kernel of Buddhism that is a part of every liv- ing creature. The Buddha-nature is the part of you that has always existed and will always exist. Your Buddha-nature is what you have in common with every other creature.

In Sanskrit, the meaning is especially instructive. Sanskrit is the founding language of Buddhism, Hinduism, and the spiritual practice of yoga. *Buddha-nature* translates as the womb containing the essence of one who has gone and returned. This reflects the belief in Bodhisattvas, creatures who have reached enlightenment, or Nirvana, and turned around to come back to this world of suffering in order to help other beings reach enlightenment. This is like a person who escapes a burning building only to run back in to save someone else. Bodhisattvas have done the hard work of reaching equanimity, but once they reach the place of mental and spiritual release, they choose instead to be born anew to lead other souls to that peace.

In 2009, while in seminary, I went to see the Dalai Lama speak at the big football stadium outside of Boston. The location was surreal: images of charging players three stories high, closed beer kiosks with pictures of women in bikinis on their signs, and Tibetan craft vendors selling singing bowls and CDs of monks chanting. The program began with the most exquisite dancing by local Boston kids of Tibetan descent, intricate dancing accompanied by unfamiliar instruments, in a huge football stadium. Everyone had cultural whiplash.

The Dalai Lama came on stage with his sweet, shy smile, in a crimson robe and a Red Sox hat, and talked about cultivating a heart of compassion not only for others but also for yourself. Practice treating yourself gently, he implored. I like this idea of practicing. So often, I feel like life skills are black or white: you have them or you don't. You have healthy self-esteem or you don't. But just practice, he said. Practice, like you would the trombone or sudoku or soccer.

A calm, holy stillness, a velvety silence, enveloped the football stadium at his words. The Dalai Lama is, even by the most secular standards, a fantastic human being. He spent most of his life negotiating with the Chinese, trying to protect his homeland of Tibet, to little effect. His people suffer, and his culture may be in its death throes. And yet he doesn't hate Chinese leaders—he loves them. He says that they are afraid. He has also been afraid; he can relate to that feeling. They are afraid, and so they grasp at power, at military might, at utter control of the Chinese and Tibetan people. They are suffering, and so they cause suffering. Just like the Israelis and Palestinians, just like the utter degradation of humanity happening at our border with Mexico. We humans are afraid, and so we hurt each other in an attempt to soothe our fear. That doesn't make it okay, he says—people should be held accountable, reparations must be made. But we can't hate our enemy, because they are just like us: afraid. Insecure. Sure they are doing it all wrong, sure that they will be called out as a fraud.

I was feeling particularly fraudulent that day. After several years of good mental health, I was having panic attacks again. The first time, I was leaving the library, satisfied to have a big paper finished. I started down the stairs, and the pit of my stomach dropped a few inches. I felt cold but began to sweat. My heart pounded, loud and much too fast. It was the reaction a person has when they are almost hit by a car, but there was no car about to hit me. What the hell?

After a bumpy start to seminary—I couldn't remember how to write a research paper, how to take notes, how to be a student—I hit my stride. Classes were hard but manageable. I had a couple of on-campus jobs, sorting mail, locking up buildings at night, so I wasn't worried about money. I had plenty of friends. Jay was still the best partner in the universe. So what the hell was up with the panic attacks?

Problem was, I was undercover with my mental illness in seminary. Sure, I was surrounded by kind, empathetic people; sure, plenty of other students were out about their health issues. But I couldn't forget the social worker who suggested I try living in a group home. I couldn't forget how many times I'd been fired because of anxiety or medication side effects. What if they knew and they kicked me out?

Do you ever feel like any moment someone will walk into your workplace and say, in an old-timey voice, "The jig is up! We found out the truth—you have no idea what you're doing. You've been faking it this whole time!" It's a waking nightmare. Somehow your friends are there too, and your parents. That high school teacher who really believed in you, that coach you admired. . . . They all look disgusted. Their faces are pulled into a repulsed grimace. Now they know you're a fraud. Now the jig is up.

I was ashamed. When I thought about coming out as mentally ill, I felt a hot welling up that started in my stomach and spread to every limb, a toxic, orange cloud of my disgust with myself. My classmates were bright and fascinating and had their shit together. How could they accept me if they knew who I really was?

The panic attacks came more and more frequently over the next few days. I wasn't sleeping, I could barely eat—my stomach rejected everything I offered it. Weak and tired, I called my doctor.

A few weeks before, I had gone to my gynecologist because my period wouldn't stop. It was usually around eight days, but eight days, ten days, two weeks, then a month had passed, and I was still menstruating. My gynecologist put me on a new form of birth control, a ring that stayed in for a month and released a low dose of hormones. I was anti–birth control then because the last time I took it, back in college, I had that whole depressive/suicidal thing for a few years. But she swore up and down that this was different, that it wouldn't impact my mood. Ha! My mood begged to differ. Down my mood zipped, crying in Target because I couldn't find the hand soap. Crying so hard I couldn't see to drive and had to pull over. Crying so hard that when I finally asked for help, my friends couldn't understand what I was saying.

Shame keeps us from seeing that we are holders of the Buddha-nature. It made me forget that no one was expecting me to be perfect. It blotted out what I knew to be true— that getting help early means less suffering, less panicking, less crying in Target. I knew that depression and anxiety were diseases and not personal failures. And yet I stuck my hand right back in that proverbial coffee cup. I made the same mistake again, ignoring symptoms and hoping they would go away. Not asking for help. Just like my niece, I repeated my error and expected a different result. I am so damn human.

The Dalai Lama says that when we make a mistake, we need to ask, "Can I love this too?" Can I love all of me, even the peevish parts? Even the insecure bits, the anxious bits? Because I can love my niece even when she sticks her hand in my cup of coffee and gets mad and hollers at me for it. It's easy. I don't expect her to be perfect. Can I extend that understanding to myself? Can I love my anxiety too? My depression too? My desire to seem like I have my shit together even when I'm freaking out? Can I love all of me?

In 1985, my faith, the Unitarian Universalist Association, adopted the Seven Principles. It was a controversial move. Some people feared that the establishment of principles would lead to a creed, that soon people would have to swear to believe the principles and vow to live by them. We like being a free-thinking tradition. But other people loved the Principles because it was a way for them to explain to non-UUs who we are. It was a list of ideas that resonate with us, ideas you could put in a brochure or on a bookmark and give to Susan at the water cooler who is always asking about your church. A very eloquent shortcut.

Those who argued for the Seven Principles felt that despite the diversity of thought among UUs, there were certain shared philosophies that needed to be crystal clear. The First Principle was the one that really won people over in all the camps. The First Principle: that every person has inherent worth and dignity.

The First Principle is still a core part of our identity as UUs, but we forget that in 1985 it was a deeply radical statement. Most of our members come from other faiths, primarily Christian faiths like Catholicism. Many heard again and again that they were bad, flawed, sinful. This Principle was a refusal to believe that any human is truly bad. Yes, we do bad things. We get scared and we screw up. But we have inherent worth. We have dignity. We can love our whole selves, not just the parts that some faiths feel are good enough.

The Buddhists and the UUs know that all humans have inherent worth and dignity. But in everyday life, I can find it hard to believe. I am so thoroughly human! And that means imperfect. But by forgiving myself for my normal human flaws, by acknowledging them and saying, "You, insecurity, I can love you too. And fear, I can love you too," I practice being kind to myself.

A week or so later, an emergency room doctor told me to take the birth control ring out. It seemed so logical after the fact—I put the hormone ring in and soon was very depressed. Why didn't it occur to me to just take it out? But talking about periods is awkward, and my gynecologist was so sure it wasn't the hormone ring, and women aren't encouraged to question authority figures, and I didn't want her to think that I didn't think she knew what she was doing. . . . (Insecurity, I can love you too. Internalized oppression, I can love you too. Even if you are a pain in my ass.) But when an official, white-coated authority told me to get off hormones, I did. I felt better the next day, and back to normal in three days.

Everyone—even hormonally weird me!—contains the Buddha-nature, a bit that is enlightened, a part that has been to Nirvana but came back to bring everyone else along. And we have bruised, sore bits too, fears and longings that aren't always expressed kindly. We are human. Will you practice being human with me? When we catch ourselves being human, we'll say, "I can love this too. I can love my broken-ness too." Let's extend to ourselves the grace we would extend to an infant who doesn't understand that sticking her fists in Aunt Kate's coffee isn't going to be pleasant. We can accept our whole selves. We can love this too.

26.

Refusing to Be Enemies

A FEW YEARS AGO I was in the Garden of Gethsemane, the wooded refuge just outside of Jerusalem to which, the Christian gospels say, Jesus retreated to pray before his trial and crucifixion. Jesus left the city to escape the throngs who were there to mark Passover at the Holy Temple and to hide from the Empire's guard. He followed a steep trail up away from the noise to a small, dark garden. It was an excellent spot to hide—from the hilltop, there is a clear view of anyone coming from the city. Jesus retreated to the garden and, the Bible says, wept tears like blood falling on the sand. Before the night was over, soldiers found him there, and he was taken away and put to death.

I too entered Gethsemane seeking refuge, not from a bloodthirsty empire bent on killing dissenters but from the unending heat emanating from the stone walls of the city and the tension that seems to electrify the very air. Jerusalem is a difficult place to visit. Jewel-toned stained glass, golden domes, glittering sand, sparkling mosaic stones— every surface is a dazzling confection for the eye. But I was there with a group of fellow ministers to study Palestinian/ Israeli relations, a human-created ugliness that seemed all the more garish in contrast to the breathtaking surroundings.

Jerusalem is a tiny desert oasis that Jews call the Promised Land, where Christians believe Jesus taught, and where Muslims have faith that the prophet Mohammad ascended to heaven to meet God. The holy home of the three monotheistic faiths, all worshipping the same God but slaughtering each other. Ancient roots of the same tree wrapped around each other, strangling. Millions of people have died staking their claim to this land, and I doubt that violence will end any time soon. The Holy Land is an exhausting, devastating place to visit, a place of glorious natural beauty and the finest art and architecture humans can create, where people inflict incredible cruelty on each other.

I needed a place to rest. I was furious with God—how can people be so terrible in God's name?—and I longed for a moment of respite to talk with her. My whole body hurt with heartache. From Jerusalem, I pictured the Garden of Gethsemane as a cool forest, shaded from the scouring sun. I imagined I would sit in the green clover and lean against an ancient oak. I can always find God in the forest. I longed to exhale the agonizing sadness that comes from visiting refugee camps and bulldozed villages, from passing through countless armed checkpoints. I dreamed of a verdant oasis safely away from the eighteen-year-old Israeli soldiers who guard every holy site and street corner in Jerusalem, baby faces contrasting painfully with the machine guns they casually cradle. The fresh holiness of new life cradling the apparatus of death.

But the Garden of Gethsemane is in the Middle East, not in my rainy home of the Pacific Northwest. It isn't greenly bursting with life but is more a sign of tenacity, a small patch of trees bravely holding ground in a dry, sandy desert. It's a plot of land the size of a small apartment complex with eight olive trees. The trees aren't tall, maybe fifteen feet, but are up to a thousand years old. They may be the oldest olive trees in the world. Not the trees Jesus wept beneath, but possibly their offspring. With elderly branches gnarled like arthritic hands, their green is of the deepest gray-black variety. Sand and scrub cover the ground, not fresh clover. The Garden of Gethsemane is a prickly ecosystem that refuses to submit to the reality of its environment. It doesn't make sense to grow here, but the desert garden isn't giving up.

In Jesus' day the garden was a remote oasis, but now it's on the itinerary of every Holy Land tourist. Expedition buses puff diesel fumes and emit guttural groans outside the garden while tourists swirl about taking photos and exclaiming in a thousand languages. There is no sitting among these trees to pray; the plot is packed with people, and the trees themselves are surrounded by metal fencing. The baby-faced military is here too, authoritatively moving the hordes past the place where Jesus sought respite and a connection with his Creator. There was no peace in the Garden of Gethsemane for me. I doubt Jesus fared any better, with his impending death and all. The Christian Bible says that Jesus begged God to find another way for his story to end. I too wanted a different story, one in which religious faith didn't lead to teenagers with machine guns, tiny children missing limbs because of hand grenades, human-caused food shortages and closed borders. I wanted to demand God rewrite the story of the Holy Land. Only I couldn't find God in that garden. I was spiritually alone in a place engorged with holy seekers. Where was God in the Holy Land?

The next day we left smoggy Jerusalem and traveled on our own fume-belching diesel bus to an agricultural community just south of Bethlehem. The city's sprawl and armed checkpoints gave way to rolling brown-green hills under a never-ending robin's egg blue sky. I felt my body relax as we stepped from the bus and smelled sage, chamomile, and marigold. A big rock painted with "We Refuse to be Enemies" in several languages marked the entrance to our destination, a farm called the Tent of Nations. We picked our way up the rocky path lined with wild herbs until we met Daoud, the Palestinian man who runs this farm and peace camp.

Daoud refuses to be enemies with anyone. He realized early in life that choosing to hate would hurt him more than it would hurt his enemy. Daoud and his family live in a series of natural caves on the farm, which has been in his family for generations. The caves are surprisingly comfortable— naturally warm in the winter and cool in the summer, with rock ledges for sitting or sleeping. A few even have solar-powered lighting. Built into rocky hillsides, they don't require drywall, insulation, or roofing. It's possible that people have dwelled in these caves for millennia.

We sat with Daoud in a bigger cave with child-painted rainbows on the walls. He served us dates and hot mint tea and told us the story of the Tent of Nations. The Nassar family has farmed the hundred acres for over a hundred years, growing grapes, olives, wheat, apricots, and almonds. In the mid-nineties, when Israeli and Palestinian relations were especially tense, Daoud decided to start holding peace camps at the farm: camps where Israeli and Palestinian children played games, learned about farming, and sang songs together. Since then the farm has added conflict resolution workshops for kids and adults, empowerment and skill-building workshops for local women, and a full load of summer camps. The aim of every program is to unite Palestinians and Israelis around common goals. Daoud wants them to meet face to face and see the goodness in each other's eyes. His guests learn to make wine, knead flatbreads, and press olive oil from the fruits of his land. They sing each other's songs, and hear each other's folktales. They leave transformed.

In 1991, the Israeli government declared the Tent of Nations Israeli state land and began the process of annexing it. The Nassar family went to court, a legal process that continues to this day. A battle of over twenty years and $170,000. In the meantime, the family has suffered through the construction of a concrete wall blocking any vehicle access to the farm and the random destruction of their property by Israeli soldiers and settlers who want to build a housing development on the land. It is a life full of hardship, and as he talked to my group we made sympathetic noises—oh, how cruel, how awful. But Daoud said, no, no, it's not cruel—they are afraid, just like we all are afraid. They want my land because they are afraid they won't have enough. No, I refuse to hate them, and you have to refuse as well. Hate, he explained, is a choice, and choosing to hate others eats up your own soul.

Not hating must take a deep discipline on Daoud's part. In May of 2014, the Israeli military showed up in the middle of the night, at 3 AM, and began to bulldoze Daoud's trees. Daoud had no legal recourse, since as a Palestinian he doesn't have rights in Israeli courts. Bulldozers dug up 1,500 apricot, olive, and apple trees, the product of twelve years of work. In the desert, growing trees is a time- and resource-intensive project. It takes at least ten years of nurturing for an olive tree to produce fruit. Trees require water, the most precious of available resources. Trees in both Israeli and Arab cultures are a sign of hope for the future. But in less than an hour, 1,500 trees were utterly destroyed. A sign of lost economy, but also a symbolic loss. Hope for the future, dismembered while Daoud and his family slept in nearby caves.

A relative recorded the destruction with his cell phone, inadvertently capturing the reaction of Daoud as well. Of course, he was devastated. He wept, like blood falling on soil, as he touched the olive tree roots ripped out of the soil. But through his tears, he said, "Father, forgive them—they don't know what they are doing."

These are the words that Jesus uttered as he lay dying on the cross: forgive them, they don't understand the pain they cause. Forgive them, they are afraid and their fear makes them cruel. Daoud is a Coptic Christian, as are many Palestinians. He said, "We refuse to hate because we believe people are created in the image of God and not meant to hurt each other. We follow the Jesus way: overcome hate and fear with kindness. We are witnesses. We are showing people how to love their neighbor as themselves."

When Daoud refuses to be enemies, he resurrects a chance for peace in the Holy Land. He resurrects his own soul. He won't forget that his fellow humans are the very image of God. He won't give into fear.

While I didn't find God in the Garden of Gethsemane, God was everywhere at the Tent of Nations. In the bright-eyed volunteers from Australia, Sweden, and Brazil who came all the way to the Holy Land to sleep on stone slabs in caves and learn about conflict resolution. In the Israeli and Palestinian women laughing through a lesson in wine making. In the busy hives of bees pollinating the fragrant herbs in harmony. But especially, God lived and breathed through Daoud and his family of hopeful farmers, loving each other and every other soul, because we are all made in the image of God.

We live in a strange age. Certainly, different tribes have warred, like the Israelis and Palestinians, since the beginning of time. The world has always been a violent place. My own country was founded on the genocide of native people. But now the whole world is our village. Now, with my smartphone, I can see the agony of our human siblings across the world—watch the children fleeing from airstrikes in Syria, old women dying of hunger in Yemen, teenage gunshot victims being carried from a US high school—in real time. How can our minds conceive of this level of sorrow? How can our hearts not break every moment? Terrible things have always happened, but now we witness nearly every loss.

The only way we survive this modern agony is together. We need a community of kind people we can grasp hold of when the grief of being alive right now threatens to sweep us away. People we can mourn with when being human is almost unbearably painful. I turn to my church family when I feel this deep sorrow and I am embraced. We light candles and sing our mourning songs, and sometimes God herself shows up to remind us that while life is often very difficult, it can also be beautiful. Especially when we see holiness in each other's faces. We practice our faith together, trying to be kind, trying to forgive, trying to be awake in the midst of suffering. We lean into our faith tradition and into each other.

Daoud lives in a country I would put on a shortlist of the most tragic places in the world. Nearly every day, his fellow humans treat him cruelly. So he clings to his family, these generations of optimistic farmers trying to eke nourishment from the sand. He practices living like Jesus in his community of Coptic Christians, knowing that he was created in the very image of God. Just like every other person, love incarnate. And because he is so well loved, his reach can extend. He can embrace the Palestinians and Israelis who come to him to learn about peacemaking. He can laugh with the adolescents awkwardly learning circle dances together, each step a move toward understanding. He can wrap them in his affection and still have room to empathize with the soldiers who bulldozed his olive trees. He can forgive them, even love them. He leans on his faith and the model set by Jesus. Because in community we can practice seeing holiness in each other, practice and practice until we see God in every face in every nation. Then we can all refuse to be enemies.

27.

A Streetcar Named Dignity

LAST SUMMER I was at a creative arts camp when I got an unwanted shoulder massage and kiss. I was in the back of the big hall during a meeting, standing by myself, when one of the camp leaders came up behind me, started aggressively massaging my shoulders, and then leaned in and kissed me on the neck. The whole thing lasted about thirty seconds before I jerked away from him and walked to the other side of the room. I felt disgusting, like my neck had been slobbered on, and small and weak, because all of this had happened without my consent. Immediately, I thought about what I was wearing, which makes me furious—I should be able to wear anything I want and not get slobbery, nonconsensual neck kisses. But the question I couldn't shake for the rest of the morning was: why me? Why did this man choose me to foist himself on? Did he think I was sending him a vibe? But I didn't even see him—he came up from behind me. How could I send a vibe if I didn't even know he was there? Like most victims, I was trying to figure out if it was my fault.

And then I remembered a family story. Like all family stories, like the Bible and the Illiad, it's been passed down orally, meaning it was told over potato salad at potlucks and Thanksgiving dinners, changed by every teller embellishing as they desired. So maybe it wasn't an exactly true story. Still, remembering it helped me make sense of my modern problem.

My great-grandmother was a night nurse at a hospital in Columbus, Ohio. She was famously thrifty and refused to take a taxi to work, even though her shift started at midnight and the big city was no place for a lady to sit around waiting for a streetcar. Mary was tough and stubborn and refused to pay for a cab just because some no-good fella might bother her. Besides, she had a sick husband at home to provide for, a consumptive man in need of medicines and treatments that ate up her nursing salary fast. Her husband's family shunned her for working on Sundays instead of going to church, but she made time-and-a-half on Sundays, and maybe if they hadn't been so busy judging her and more interested in helping her with the bills, she wouldn't have had to work on the Lord's Day. In fact, at Mary's age, she should have been retired; she was the oldest nurse at the hospital. But bills needed to be paid, so she pulled on her white nurse's dress and snow boots and walked to the streetcar stop.

It was a cold winter's night, snow flurries flying without making an impression. It was midwinter and snow had lost its romantic quality, heaped up in gray-brown piles by the side of every road. Mary was at the streetcar stop waiting, pushing down her glove periodically to check her thin-chained watch, the watch my mother has now. She had on a long wool coat in some practical color, something dark to mask wear and tear, and a tiny pocketbook over her shoulder. This is the important part of the story: the pocketbook. A small purse with just a tissue, the streetcar fare, a tube of lipstick, and (depending on the teller) half of a ham and cheese sandwich. The sandwich was added so that the storyteller could remark on how Mary ate like a bird and had a tiny bird body to match—under one hundred pounds, wrists like a child's, hardly ate a thing. An important detail because as Mary waited for the streetcar, a large man passed by and grabbed her purse and took off running.

I'm betting this fellow thought grabbing a tiny elderly woman's purse was an easy way to make a few dollars, but Mary wouldn't let go of her pocketbook. He tried to run down the street, but he found that he was dragging the purse with Mary tripping along with him. A crowd gathered to watch the odd sight—not one brave soul intervening, but plenty of commentary. Folks yelling at Mary to let go of the purse: "You fool, let him have it before he hurts you!" and others yelling at the would-be purse snatcher, "Leave her alone, creep!" It was a divided crowd, women hollering at the thief, men hollering at Mary. There were probably plenty of household arguments that evening. After a few tense minutes, Mary slipped, falling on her back on the ice. She still didn't release the bag but inadvertently pulled the thief down on top of her arm, breaking it with a loud crack. The man looked her in the eyes, yelled, "Dang stubborn woman!" and released the purse, running and sliding off into the night.

By then, the streetcar had arrived. The driver jumped out to help Mary up, asking, "What was in that pocketbook?" I suppose he thought it must be stuffed with rubies, or at least some token worth great emotional weight—a lock of a dead lover's hair, something sentimental. At this point, Mary had snapped open her purse to make sure nothing was lost, and the driver looked in, noting the humble goods. He was shocked at the nothing she had fought so hard for, asking, "Why didn't you just let go?"

Mary huffed, "And reward that kind of behavior? Let ruffians think they can take what they like with no consequences?" Her arm hanging at an odd angle, she refused an ambulance, citing the expense, and took the streetcar to the hospital to have her arm set.

Growing up, I thought this story was about the power of being stubborn, the ability to beat the bad guys with tenacity, the importance of women standing up to male bullies. Refusing to be a victim. Realizing that even though justice demands a price, it is worth it. But when I brought it up with my mom recently, she gave me that familiar "Did I raise a crazy person?" look. "I told you that story so you would learn about choosing your battles. You were always so worked up about every little thing, I wanted you to know that one metaphorical pocketbook wasn't worth breaking an arm over."

Family stories matter, even when they are only partly true. They are the myths that tell us how we are supposed to behave in the world. They can make us proud of our clan. In a family with a significant history of mental illness, having stories about resilience remind me that we aren't just people with depression. That day, standing in the big hall at camp, the story reminded me that I had a choice. I could fight back like Mary or take my mom's advice and let it go. Either way, I was a Landis woman and I was strong enough and smart enough to make my own decision.

In the Unitarian Universalist tradition we live by Seven Principles, and the first Principle is that every person has inherent worth and dignity. Inherent worth means that our value can't be taken away by how other people treat us. When that man roughly massaged and kissed me, I felt like I didn't have control of my own autonomy. I felt like my worth and dignity were being ignored so that he could get a cheap thrill. I wasn't okay with that.

I reported him to a member of the board of directors, Amy, who said four essential things that I try to remember in case I am ever in her shoes. These four things changed the way I thought about the situation and gave me my power back. They were:

1. I believe you.
2. It is not your fault.
3. It isn't okay that he did that and it shouldn't have happened.
4. I am going to make sure there are repercussions so that he knows it isn't okay and so that hopefully he won't do it to anyone else.

It isn't easy to remember our worth and dignity. Maybe we have been told that we are worthless and that we don't deserve autonomy. Maybe our desires have been ignored so many times that we don't know how to say no. But my UU faith reminds me that I matter, just like you get to matter. We all have value. We are each a precious soul in a holy body, and we deserve respect. We deserve respect even when it upsets the status quo or means reporting abuse by a popular leader.

If someone has violated you, I believe you. It isn't your fault. It isn't okay that it happened—it breaks my heart that someone would hurt precious you—and it shouldn't have happened. I hope that you can find a safe person in your life who can help you make sure it doesn't happen again. You can choose if you want to press charges—it is your decision, you are strong and smart enough to make it on your own, and you aren't obligated to either report it or to let it go to avoid causing drama. (Unless you are a required reporter, in which case you have to report it to protect other people. Sorry.)

Guidelines like the Seven Principles remind us of who we are and what we believe. In times of great difficulty, they are worth more than gold. Family stories fill much the same role. They give us strength when strength is in short supply. Even though many generations of my family have suffered with severe mental illness, we are resilient. We are night nurses supporting sick husbands, rebels who befriended Japanese Americans during a war with Japan, kind folks who volunteer to build the church's pews, who live close to the land. And unfortunately or fortunately, depending on your perspective, people who are stubborn enough to get an arm broken over a pocketbook containing a lipstick, bus fare, a tissue, and maybe half of a sandwich.

28.

Good Guys

"UNCLE JAY is nice to people who no one else will be nice to, for his job," I explained to our niece, who understandably looked confused.

"Why isn't anyone nice to them?" she asked, all big brown eyes and blonde ponytail. In her world, "not nice" is something that happens on episodes of *Sesame Street*, when a different-looking monster moves to the neighborhood and the other residents make fun of him. People not being nice is a fictional problem that is resolved in thirty minutes with hugging and learning that "different is good!" at the end.

How do I explain that her Uncle Jay spends his days with formerly homeless men who struggle with the fun cocktail of schizophrenia and dementia, plus an extra dash of either trauma, cognitive delays, brain damage from drug use, or PTSD from homelessness? I can't see telling my niece that no one is nice to these guys because they talk to themselves, because they yell at creatures no one else can see. Because their dialogue is all nonsense, because they think the FedEx guy is sending them telepathic messages to eat the batteries in the phone. Because some of them are violent and addicted, would do anything—mug a nun—if it meant getting a cigarette.

I don't know how to explain mental illness, systemic poverty, or generational trauma to a three-year-old. I don't know how to explain that for one dollar above minimum wage, my husband tries to convince grown men not to leave their group homes because they feel safer living on the street. I'm not sure how to explain that the men have medicine that makes the voices they hear go away, but they don't trust it. They fear it is poisoned or that it eliminates their special psychic powers, or they don't believe they need it. Uncle Jay tries to talk them into taking it. I think the only part of the job she understands is that Uncle Jay's clients don't want to take showers, so he tries to talk them into bathing for the good of their housemates. My niece hates bathing but understands the problems of stinkiness.

My niece is unfortunately not losing interest in this conversation, unlike yesterday when I tried to explain feminism to her and she started banging her head on a wall for entertainment. But I recall that she does know the Bible—her parents are Jehovah's Witnesses, and they are serious about Biblical literacy. So we talk about Jesus.

"You know the Good Samaritan?" I ask.

"Yes!" She responds. "Bullies were mean to him and beat him up. People aren't supposed to hit each other, but sometimes they do anyway. But not me because I'll get a time-out. But bullies were mean to him and beat him up, so the Good Samaritan had to help him. Even though the guy thought Samaritans were bad guys, they were good guys really. And the guys he thought were good were really bad, 'cause they didn't help."

This kid is a theological genius. She should be teaching in a seminary.

"So Uncle Jay is like the Good Samaritan, and he helps people who are sick get better."

"Like a doctor?" she asked.

"Like a doctor for your head," I replied.

Later I have to squelch a laugh when she goes up to Jay, puts his hand on her head, and asks if it feels healthy. He looks so confused. But Jay's job is hard to explain and hard to understand, if only because understanding it means having to acknowledge that there is a whole class of people, homeless and mentally ill, who suffer for years before dying, often at a young age. His job requires looking at reality harder than I prefer to. This is a reality that really sucks. His clients make me doubt God, the goodness of God.

People think that since I am a minister, I am the designated good person in Jay's and my relationship. But they are way off—being a minister is fun. I hold babies, bless animals, receive dozens of hugs. I sit on the floor to sing songs with kids. I talk to a captive audience for an hour every week—talk about an ego boost! I visit people in the hospital, which sounds sad, but most of the time I am awed by their resiliency. And by the gentle care of medical professionals, who aren't clergy but do holy work. I go to rallies and protests where I am buoyed by my fellow citizens' passion for justice. My job is pretty fun. And sometimes people leave cookies in the church kitchen.

Jay is definitely the good person in our relationship, which has been the case since we met. The first time I asked him out, he said he couldn't because he was painting the local domestic violence shelter with other volunteers from his church all weekend. I nearly fainted from lust. He, like my brother, Tom, is always quietly helping people, quietly pitching in with no desire for recognition. Being a minister is doing the occasional good thing and getting loads and loads of praise for it. Jay does loads and loads of good things and hopes no one notices.

I think Jay is my *beshert*, the one God paired me with. It's a Jewish concept, that every person has another half they are meant to spend life with. It goes against all my theologies of free will to believe in having a beshert, but who said love was logical? Jay says that he loves me too, but he thinks God has bigger problems than who I fall in love with.

Still, there is a holiness to our union. I met Jay at a Unitarian Universalist retreat, and we were friends for a few years while I recovered from my divorce from Drew. Just friends, no funny business. Maybe that is why our bond is so gentle—we started as buddies, with no lust to muck things up. Jay is an agnostic UU, which means he believes in kindness and not trying to pin God down. God is too big for just one idea, after all. I think that is why he can do the difficult work that he does: he doesn't expect reasons from God. He doesn't demand answers to the big question of why his clients have to endure so much suffering. He just quietly helps them cope without looking for a grand, philosophical meaning.

My Jewish colleagues talk about a cool concept, *tikkun olam*, which means to heal the world. The idea is that we humans partner with God to heal all that is hurting. My favorite part is that this partnership doesn't mean we have to do all the fixing ourselves: we are partnering with God and all of humanity. So often, I feel like my small deeds don't really matter because there is so much suffering. Tikkun olam reminds me that I am not in the world-healing business alone. Jay embraces tikkum olam by helping his clients without getting bogged down by all the systemic injustice he can't overturn. One person at a time, one conversation at a time, healing happens. Tikkun olam, one soul at a time.

My niece the theologian probably could explain all of this better than I can. An hour or so after our conversation about Uncle Jay, she came up to me and said, "You know, sometimes the bad guys need help too. Even though they are bad." Her uncle and I try to remember that, and that every little bit of the world we can heal is part of our partnership with God.

29.

Ferocious Love

I WAS WALKING along a dirt trail overlooking the vast ocean. Huge waves crashed mercilessly onto rocky cliffs. A tiny fishing boat, red with blue and white trim, whooshed up and down on the white foam, seeming much too small for the swells that erupted from the deep. They created mountains of water that quickly bottomed out into deep bowls, the boat staying upright despite the impossible physics of steep angles and rapid movement. The utter chaos of nature that is the everyday reality of the northern coast of Spain.

Safely on my perch, occasionally doused with salty spray but otherwise secure, I walked as slowly as I could stand to. Our spiritual guide kept reminding us: if you usually walk slowly, try walking quickly. If you usually walk quickly, go slowly. Every day, my group of twenty pilgrims on the Norte route of the Camino de Santiago set off together.

Quickly the group separated, with a retired hospice chaplain and farmer from South Dakota, eighty-two years old, taking the lead. She was so fast I was surprised her hiking boots didn't spark as she walked.

I strolled along behind her, looking at every unusual flower, leaf, or colorful mushroom, singing under my breath unconsciously. Our guru had said, "If you walk fast, walk slow." Looking right at our eighty-something retired chaplain, she added, "The first should be last, finishing up today, and the last first." Our speed demon rolled her eyes and walked fast anyway, but I am a teacher pleaser, and if the guide said to walk slowly, I was going to walk slowly.

I tried walking meditation, focusing on the feel of the muscles in my feet rolling along the ground. I smelled the greenness of the meadow. I heard the birds, singing different songs than back home, and much louder. And the sea rollicked along. I was mindful, I was aware, I wasn't thinking of the future or the past. For about thirty seconds, anyway. And then the grief crashed in.

It was the ocean that got me. Or the swooping gulls, or the tiny, perfect, purple wildflowers. It was all so beautiful that it hurt. I was falling in wild and passionate love with the earth and then I remembered: it's all burning. Climate change, extinction, the world on fire. Naomi, my tiny niece, one year old, inheriting the smoky air and chemical-laden water and a climate where crops burn off their stems before fruiting and fields flood too often for animals to graze—and there is nothing to feed those animals anyway. Overcrowding in the center of nations as coastal cities like New York, Boston, Mumbai, Seattle, and Bangkok flood more and more frequently until they are completely underwater. Violence against climate refugees and violence due to food shortages.

We have ten years to cut emissions in half, just to slow this planetary catastrophe down, and our president wants to allow more fuel emissions. The new president of Brazil wants to trade the Amazon, the world's biggest safehold of carbon, for quick cash. Inadvertently, my pace quickened on the trail, my chest constricted, my blood raced through my veins. "I won't live long enough to get old," I thought. "And today's children suffer like no generation has suffered, even more than the Greatest Generation in the brutal trenches of a world war. They will die alongside the orcas and polar bears, alongside the bees and butterflies, suffering and then disappearing."

Grief. Horror. Shame. It swelled up higher than the waves tossing the fishing boat and then plunged me into a deep bowl of despair. I checked in with God.

For me, God is the relationship between living creatures. How I treat you, how you treat me. This is the God who is always developing, always changing. The God of process theology, of cause and effect. The God who dwells among us, anywhere there is life and nowhere there is not. I feel God's presence best in wild places: along the shore, on dirt paths. So I called out to this God of my understanding—what the hell should we do? What can we do?

The great theologian Anne Lamott says that all prayers fit into one of three categories: Help, Thanks, or Wow. When I think about the climate catastrophe, all my prayers are Help. Help! I feel completely powerless. Seventy percent of carbon emissions are caused by one hundred companies, all of whom are well connected politically. Does it matter if I compost my potato peels? A tiny bit. But without billions of dollars, how can I create change? Help! I don't want all that I love to perish. Help! These amazing children can't have been born just to suffer. Help!

Once in a while, maybe every five or so years, I get a pretty clear communication from the universe, or God, or the wisdom that lives inside of me that I can't access as often as I would like. Maybe it's my ancestors—sometimes the voice sounds just like my grandmother. Maybe it is the earth herself, and when I get quiet enough, I can hear the wisdom she is continually sharing. That day the message was loud and clear. It was, "Keep walking."

What? Keep walking? I was on the Camino, in a pasture above the ocean—what choice did I have? Or course I was going to keep walking. Could you be more specific? "Keep walking," I grumbled. "Thank you, Captain Obvious." But I put one foot down, then the other, and soon I noticed the muscles in my feet rolling along. The smell of green leaves in the sun. The birds singing their loud, unfamiliar song. Soon

I was in love with the earth again. And in that love, there was resilience. In that love was the courage to continue.

Joanna Macy, the environmental activist, Buddhist, and ecofeminist, teaches that to preserve the planet, we must fiercely love the planet. She writes that if your child has leukemia, you don't say, "Oh well, I am not going to go to your bedside, I'm not going to spend time with you—it's too sad." If your mother is dying, you don't stop loving her. But somehow we feel that we can't face climate destruction because it is so painful. The reality of it is too agonizing. And so we turn away. But that fierce love, that ferocious love that parents have for their children—even if their children are very sick, even if they may die, causing the parents unimaginable grief—is what will sustain us in this climate crisis. It will keep us from drowning in hopelessness as we face countless obstacles: multinational corporations, governments big and small, your quirky aunt who thinks climate change is a hoax. Ferocious love will lead us to defend the earth. We can abandon despair and love this world like it deserves to be loved. Not out of fear, or guilt, or grief. Out of courageous, fierce love.

We don't live in a culture that embraces difficult feelings. We aren't taught to sit with sadness and pain but to drive it away. We are so terrified of grief that we numb ourselves with booze or TV or busyness—busyness most of all. We run around doing a thousand essential things until we are too weary to feel our anguish. But sorrow is a part of our human experience. It is necessary. If we are numb, we aren't really alive, and this wonderful, terrible world that we were mysteriously born into, which we will exit in just as much mystery, is wasted on us. The bright green smell of a prairie in the summer and the symphony of birdsong. When we numb ourselves, we miss all of it, the pain and the beauty.

It is easy to let busyness take over. Don't do it. Reject numbness; feel the pleasure and the pain. When you feel the pain of climate sorrow, sit with it. Notice where it lives in your body. Don't push it away. Wait for it to transform. Your anguish becomes your strength. It becomes ferocious love.

Humanity has caused tremendous harm to this planet. Some can be slowed, a little can be reversed. Some is not repairable. Some species will not be recovered. Some life is gone forever. But our Buddhist eco-activist Joanna Macy says that she was moved to begin her environmental activism when she realized that the decisions made now, decisions made with profit as the main motivator, had consequences reaching into geological time. Meaning that not just the next generation will be impacted by this climate crisis but generations for thousands of years. Geological time is so hard to fathom. We are impacting not just the next generation or the next ten but the lives of creatures far, far into a future beyond what we can imagine. So we must love life—all creatures, great and small—with such ferocity that our grief turns to strength. Like a parent with a sick child, we are not consumed by our sadness at the present and future suffering. We hold our grief and watch it transform into a mighty and powerful love that will not be stopped until every generation is safe.

30.

Heaven Is a Place
on Earth

Around Thanksgiving, I was packing up to leave for
the day when a woman I didn't know called the church.
Her voice was hard to make out. She was crying, in that
choking way that garbles your voice. She said she was looking for a place for her mother. For her mother to . . . ? I
thought maybe they needed to have a memorial for their
mother, or she was looking for an assisted living referral,
but she said no, it's harder than that. It's stranger than that.

She said, "I can't say it—can you call my brother?"
I penciled down the local number and thought, "How did I
get into all this?" I called her brother. He was teary too. He
said that their mother had attended an event at the church,
a concert or something; he couldn't remember the details.
Anyway, she thought our church was beautiful, she thought

what we believed was beautiful. That was a year or two ago, and now she was in her nineties, in assisted living in a place nearby, and she was really suffering. She was in constant pain, unrelenting agony; nothing could relieve it. And she wanted to die.

In Washington and a handful of other states, people can petition the court for the right to choose the time they depart this life. A person has to be very ill, usually very old, and in sound mental health to be approved. So this woman went through the long and complicated authorization process and got the go-ahead: yes, you may end your life. But her nursing home, a Catholic institution, wouldn't allow her to swallow the handful of pills that constitutes assisted suicide. She wanted to go to her son's home, just blocks from here, but he lives in an old apartment building that isn't handicapped accessible, and she couldn't sit upright, much less walk up the stairs. So Compassionate Choices, the nonprofit who managed this Death with Dignity procedure, said the other option was a cheap motel, the kind that rented by the hour, the kind that wouldn't ask questions about all the medical equipment that would need to be hauled in, wouldn't care what was going on. But her son said this was just too sad—yeah, they didn't have any money, but did that mean that their mom had to die in a cheap motel room?

So he called us. The social worker representing Compassionate Choices said he had never heard of euthanasia happening in a church, but he didn't think it could hurt to ask. "So . . . ," the son paused and took a deep breath. "So I guess I am calling . . . to ask if my mom can . . . well, die in your church. She really likes you," he rushed in, "you mean something to her, even if you don't know her. . . ."

We talked for a while. The procedure needed to happen soon because his mom was in agony, pain crushing her body every second. He explained that if we were willing to open our space to this procedure, a nurse and a social worker would come and administer the medicine. That his mother would arrive in a medicab and a hearse would take away her body. That he and his siblings would be there in her final moments. That the procedure would take between two and four hours. That all they needed from us was space— a place for his mom to make this last choice.

I didn't commit either way, just let him know I would call him back and hung up the phone. I had so many emotions, but first, sadness for his mother's suffering. Anger that natural death wouldn't come for this elderly woman in constant pain but did take away babies in the NICU and happy twenty-somethings with cancer. Death was close at hand for a young man in the congregation whose cello playing brought us all to tears, who was gentle and kind and had two small children. But no, death couldn't take this elderly lady instead, this woman who was so ready to go.

I felt confusion over my role in these strangers' lives. I don't even know these people! I closed my office door and sat on the floor—when the world is spinning uncontrollably, when there are literally life and death decisions to make, I find that meditating is the only way to slow life down to a manageable speed. And in meditation I found that I kept coming back to my anger: why me? I'm not proud of this, but, to be really honest, I kept thinking: why did they have to call me? I am in my very first year of ministry, I haven't written Sunday's sermon yet, I am already this close to overwhelmed. Why a huge moral decision like this when I am so unprepared?

It's not pretty, but it's what I was thinking in those panicked first moments. Fortunately, a greater force prevailed. A deep source of universal wisdom, available to any who seek a cosmic truth: Facebook. I remembered that a friend had posted a Thomas Merton quote online that morning, a bit of wisdom that was just what I needed. Merton, our modern American mystic and monastic, said, "Our job is to love others without stopping to inquire whether or not they are worthy. That is not our business, and in fact, it is nobody's business. What we are asked to do is love, and this love itself will render both ourselves and our neighbors worthy, if anything can."

Ahh yes, love. Love, the reason we do church. Yep, I don't know this woman at all. I don't know whether she is worthy, whatever that means. But my job in this life is to love her. My job is to love her at this moment when she is so fragile, so vulnerable, so in need of love.

In my life, I have received this big, engulfing, no-questions-asked love. From old church ladies who winced at my blue hair but loved me anyway; from my "Do we have to talk about feelings?" little brother when I was shattered into depressed, weeping shards on the kitchen floor and he sat beside me. From seminary friends after I told them, terrified, that I wondered if a person with my mental health history could be—should be—a minister, and they said, "Hell yes!" From church board members after I shoved my foot halfway down my throat, from nurses in the psych ward—I am broken yet beloved. In all the moments when I needed love but didn't deserve it, hadn't earned it, couldn't appreciate it—love enveloped me, a bounty without end.

I saw this bounty in my congregation. Fearless, unshakeable love for each of this world's broken souls. It's why I fell in love with them. Every Sunday we say, "Whoever you are, wherever you came from, whoever you love, wherever you are on life's journey—you are welcome here." It knocks the wind right out of me. I didn't know the human heart could hold so much love before I met this congregation.

Was my congregation's love big enough to house this biggest of transitions, this move from our reality into the great mystery, for this fragile woman? Could we embrace this stranger without stopping to inquire if she was worthy? We didn't know what she believed in, how she lived, if she was kind or cruel. We didn't know how she voted or if she was a good parent. We had to embrace our own First

Principle: she had inherent worth and dignity. Not because she did or was anything; she was born precious and holy. So with that in mind, we would help usher her out of this life. Yes, I thought then, and I deeply believe now, yes—our love is big enough to include this stranger.

I emailed the board with "Urgent-SOS" in the subject line and told them just that: this woman needs shelter, she needs a place to die, and I think we should be that shelter. Our love is big enough, our love is strong enough. I asked, "What do you think?" Reflecting now, I think this must have been a heck of an email to receive at work, in the midst of a busy day. Hey, is it okay if this woman that we've never met comes to the church to take some life-ending drug cocktail? Hey, can you put aside all your complicated feelings about life and death and think over this super weird, no-precedent question that literally determines if an elderly stranger, suffering in unimaginable agony, can end her life in our airy, bright sanctuary or has to go to a by-the-hour roach motel? And no, I don't know if the press will get word of this, I don't know if there will be protestors. No, there is no legal precedent; yes, we could be sued. And please let me know by 5 PM.

The board quickly and unequivocally agreed: the congregation's love is great enough to encompass this suffering woman. This is our chance, several members said, to walk our talk. Several years ago, many congregants advocated for Death with Dignity legislation. They went door to door;

they worked phone banks. "This is our chance to live what we believe," they said. "This is what we learned in our faith community: to love other people without stopping first to see if they are worthy."

And so, the week before Christmas, on a chilly afternoon with the weak winter sun shining, an ambulance brought a suffering older woman to our church. A nurse wheeled her tiny body inside on a hospital stretcher. Her children nestled her into a bed with familiar worn-soft linens and her favorite quilt. Pictures of family surrounded her, sunlight slipped in the back windows, and her son and daughter held her as she took first some antinausea medicine and then an hour later drank a concoction that ushered her into sleep and then death. A nurse, a social worker, and her children were present. I waited next door, out of the way but available. Within that second hour I saw the hearse arrive, and her son walked over, red-eyed but smiling, to tell me she was gone peacefully on her way.

"Our job is to love others without stopping to inquire whether or not they are worthy." I am grateful that my church family taught me radical love—love strong enough to shelter a stranger. To let her last act be a deliberate one. It's a strength I wouldn't have without religious community. It is too easy for me to focus strictly on myself, to be the center of my own universe. Part of this is social media, part of it is the human ego, some of it is that we live less communal lives than ever before in history. From birth we are angled to gaze only inward. Life in spiritual community is a corrective to that self-centeredness. I spend an hour a week in the sanctuary, and I am reminded that I am one being among billions and that through the great questions of faith, we are connected. Why are we here? Why do we die? Why does this life matter? We search for meaning together, and as a side effect our self-absorption is reduced. As a side effect, we recall that we are called to love others without first inquiring as to whether they are worthy. And even if we ourselves are not worthy (because God knows I am not), in spiritual community we get to experience that tidal wave of love wash over us. Broken but so loved.

I don't know what will happen when I die. I have no creed regarding the great beyond. But here in this reality, my life is deeper, kinder, and more interesting because I am a part of a congregation. A chance to think deeply about life's big questions alongside people older and younger, whom I have grown to love, brings me back every Sunday morning, despite how late the concert went last night, despite my friends inviting me to brunch, despite my love of sleeping late. Spiritual community gives my life a shape and a meaning greater than just me thinking about myself. The chance to be loved not for who I am, but sometimes despite who I am. I don't know if there is a heaven, but the blessing of spiritual community is paradise right here, on this earth.

31.

Riding Horses
to Heaven

Saint-Jean-Pied-de-Port was so perfectly charming, so flawlessly French that it felt like watching a Disney holiday movie, the sort where an everyday American girl falls in love with a dashing European stable boy only to learn that he is really a prince. Was this a real place? I stumbled, dazed, along cobblestone streets in the tiny village, past the ancient stone castle surrounded by green pine trees that fronted the blue Pyrenees, only a few shades darker than the blue sky. As people nodded hello to me with a "Buen Camino," I was startled into remembering that they could see me too—this wasn't a film, but a real idyll, a Shangri-La tucked into the mountains that form the border of Spain and France.

Alabaster-painted stone houses with either red or forest green wooden shutters lined the road, their window boxes full of bright geraniums. French children practiced the skipping, hopping movements of Morris dance in the schoolyard, wearing crisp uniforms and singing loudly and unself-consciously. Women walked arm-in-arm, carrying loaves of fresh bread; men smoked endless cigarettes outside at tiny café tables while slurping even tinier cups of espresso and gesticulating broadly. Were all the French stereotypes real?, I wondered, as a family on horseback trotted by.

The train from Toulouse had been packed with fellow wannabe pilgrims ready to start the Camino de Santiago, the ancient walking route that spiritual seekers tread from the French-Spanish border in the high Pyrenees to Santiago, on the western coast of Spain. Around 500 miles on foot, through tiny villages and a few big cities, the whole route takes around thirty-five days. Like me, most Americans do only a portion. We get laughingly few vacation days compared to the Europeans, as they never failed to remind us. In Saint-Jean-Pied-de-Port, the starting line, we were from all over the world but nearly identical: huge, brightly colored backpacks, tan hiking boots, eager to compare walking routes over the mountains and blister remedies.

The Saint-Jean leg was rumored to be the most brutal leg of the Camino. There was the route over the mountains, fifteen miles long and in places straight up, more like climbing a ladder than walking. Then there was an easier route along the highway, but Camino veterans claimed it was much more dangerous because of the huge trucks careening alongside the slim shoulder. But at least, I thought in the back of my mind, if you give up on the highway route you can hail a cab. There was no giving up on the mountain; the trail went higher than any road.

My stomach roiled with nerves as I left the train and, hefting my pack, checked the map for the best route to my albergue. An albergue is a hostel but just for Camino pilgrims, and nearly all pilgrims stay in them. They are much cheaper than a hotel, and it is reassuring to bunk with people who don't think you are senseless for taking on this arduous journey. In the albergue you don't have to explain why you want to walk the Camino. I was eager to avoid that question because I didn't know why. I trained for a year, researched gear, bought special socks, and flew across the world. All that was easy compared to considering why I was walking.

I was on a six-month sabbatical from ministry, and I felt dry. On my best days, preparing for worship felt like turning on the faucet—I opened my heart and the Spirit poured through. Sometimes the faucet was stuck, some days the water only trickled, but on the best days it gushed through me and into the congregation. It didn't feel effortless by any means, but it also wasn't solitary. I wasn't alone. While I can't pin down what this Spirit is that moves through me—

the Christian Holy Spirit or the Buddha-nature or the tempestuous Muse—that doesn't make it any less real.

When the water only trickled, I still had all my seminary learning up my sleeve. I could talk about the Hebrew etymology of this or that word, or talk about the historical context of the foundations of Islam and how it was influenced by Judaism. Sure, it wasn't spiritually invigorating for the congregation, but at least it was interesting. Good information for a cocktail party or a pub quiz night. It wasn't the kind of preaching I wanted to do—sermon by way of academic lecture—but sometimes it was all I had. But after six years of ministry, I was out of smart-sounding filler. The congregation knew all of my fun facts about how the Hebrew Bible's Genesis echoed Assyrian legend and the real reasons the Catholic church split into Roman and Greek Orthodox. More terrifying, the holy faucet was trickling more often than it was gushing. I loved being a minister, but I feared I was out of ministry to share. What if the Spirit was done with me?

I told my therapist I was walking the Camino in order to open myself up to the Holy. To get really quiet so I could hear divine wisdom. But it was more like I was hunting down the Spirit. On this pilgrimage trail, walked by holy seekers for centuries before the Catholics claimed it as the Way of Saint James in 842, I would find God if I had to climb every damn mountain to do so. I would fight blisters the size of an adult thumb, demanding at every step that God show me her face. Ten years earlier I had obeyed a holy call to ministry, upending my life and Jay's too. I moved across the country twice. I was slowly paying down a gigantic student loan. I had jumped in faith first, and I wasn't letting God leave me now. I kept going back to the Biblical story of Jacob wrestling the angel, refusing to let go until the angel blessed him. I was getting my blessing if I had to walk the length of Spain to do so.

This isn't the most peaceful way to approach God. As a teenager I had the verse "Be still and know that I am God" posted on my desk, but the reality has always been more like me demanding and whining and hollering until God, probably with a holy eye roll, acquiesces. This probably has to do with my genetic predisposition toward being a stubborn and impatient ass and my anxiety disorder. Anxiety disorder feels like I know the whole world is crumbling—I can see the earth shaking and the sky falling—but all around me, everyone is going about their business like all is well. And it makes no sense because I can feel my heart galloping and my stomach flip-flopping and every nerve is screaming, "Run!" So while other religious folks are sitting in silent meditation or singing Taizé chants, I am yelling, "God! Yeah, you! I know you can hear me! Get down here!"

This is how I found myself in the perfectly lovely town of Saint-Jean-Pied-de-Port on the French border, while children did Morris dances and Frenchmen drank wine, and in my heart I hollered "I'm coming for you" at God while looking for the pilgrim hostel for which I had prepaid €6. I found it (the hostel, not God) on a perfect green hill, across from a pasture of perfect, golden horses whose muscles rippled in the late-afternoon sunlight. A little boy was outside of the old stone house, stalking an annoyed kitten through the flowerbeds while chickens clucked in a pen. As I approached, he yelled "Peregrino! Peregrino!" and streaked into the house. His beautiful mother came out and helped me find a bunk in the garage-turned-albergue. Then she invited me to sit on the porch and drink wine, because apparently that is what people do in the afternoon in France, besides smoking cigarettes and buying bread.

As we talked, the little boy reappeared and was introduced as Michel. Michel, being the child of hostel owners and all of four years of age, spoke perfect French, English, German, and Spanish and was eagerly learning Italian. He was disappointed to learn that I had no Italian to teach him and appalled when I admitted to only speaking English. "Only English?" he cried, as if I had told him that I had four tails covered with oozing warts. "Only English?" he cried until his mother gave him that universal look all mothers have that means "Be quiet now or else."

Despite my obvious language-related failings, I was the only pilgrim currently available to him, and so he decided I was worthy of a visit to his treehouse, an architecturally questionable structure teetering above the chicken pen. Calling me "only English," he took my hand and led me to the ladder. As we climbed, he chattered on in excellent English and once in the little room introduced me, one by one, to his collection of half-broken toys. It was a motley assortment of dolls with one eye missing and stuffed animals with the fur rubbed off. In my American-ness, I noticed that he didn't have a single toy gun or soldier, a lovely surprise. Even at church we have the occasional toy gun sneak into a Sunday School classroom, even in peace-loving Seattle.

Michel pulled a purple plastic horse from the pile and said, "We will ride this horse to heaven to see my Grand-mère. It isn't too far if we ride the horse."

"When did your Grand-mère go to heaven?" I asked gently, aware that Michel's joyful mood had shifted into something more reflective.

"This summer. I miss her. I want to go visit her, but Maman says I can only go in my heart. Wait, we can take this train!" he said, pulling a modern-looking train car from the pile. "That will be even faster!"

"My Grand-mère died last year too. Sometimes it makes me feel really sad, because I miss her so much."

"What do you do?"

"I close my eyes and remember the times we were together. She used to let me eat cucumbers right from her garden. We went swimming a lot. She was almost always laughing, and when she laughed, her eyes and forehead scrunched up and she tipped her head back. When I think about her, it's like she is right here with me."

I paused, realizing that words like "cucumber" and "scrunched" might be unfamiliar to Michel, but when I looked over, he had his eyes closed and was smiling dreamily. We sat silently for a few minutes, Michel unself-conscious and turned in toward his memories. I listened to the chickens below and thought about my grandmother's huge backyard vegetable patch and how familiar the sounds of hens clucking would be to her. I thought about how she always seemed proud of my far-flung travels, despite her own clucking that it was best to stay close to home. I reveled in the sweetness hidden in the bittersweet aching of memories of a time that would never come again. What joy we had shared. How my grandmother had lavished love on me, a bounty of hugs and kisses and words. Every day a feast of embraces. Thank you, Goddess, for that joy. And then, suddenly, Michel's mother was calling him to set the table, and our treehouse adventure was over.

That night, lying in my bunk in the hostel, listening to the snuffles and murmurs of the other pilgrims, I worried about my future. What if I couldn't find God? What if my spiritual faucet was permanently turned off? And as clearly as if she was in the room, I heard my grandmother say "Katharine Yvonne" (she always insisted on using my full name), "why do you worry so much? The sun will rise without you fretting over it." I silently laughed with her and agreed. I could nearly feel her cheek, skin soft as a bird's feather, as she pressed her papery lips to my forehead in farewell.

I remembered Michel's happily contemplative face in the silent treehouse, how God danced across his small features, resurrecting his grand-mère, if only for a few moments. Maybe God wasn't so hard to find after all. As soon as I stopped demanding, she was there, in the comforting of a new friend and in quietly recalling memories of Grandma. In the pine trees and high, blue Pyrenees. And with those thoughts, I fell asleep.

32.

Spiritual Safety Rails

THE NEXT DAY I climbed the Pyrenees. Lest that sound terribly brave and adventurous, the Pyrenees are only around 9,000 feet high, tiny compared to Everest (29,029) or even the Rockies (14,440). And I was climbing them with roughly 700 other pilgrims, a sputtering, breathless line of souls wondering why the hell this had seemed like a good idea when they were planning it on their couch back home. For the most part, we weren't the athletic "Let's hike the Appalachian Trail before breakfast" type. The Camino isn't really tough enough to draw that crowd. While a day's walk can be fifteen to twenty miles, it is mostly flat, and the well-spaced villages mean pilgrims can walk five miles, have a coffee and pastry break, walk another five and stop for a sit-down lunch, then walk five and stop for a glass of delicious local wine. But the first leg, from Saint-Jean to Roncesvalles, included a great deal of elevation gain. There aren't many places to rest, and there is a constant pressure to hurry in order to arrive at the monastery hostel in Roncesvalles before dark, when a pilgrim is likely to get lost in the forest. The first leg is the worst leg, we heard over and over again, but if you finish it you know you can handle every other leg of the Camino. A sentiment that would probably seem more comforting on the other side of the mountains.

I woke up to the rooster crowing and Michel's mom swearing back at it. Most of the other pilgrims were awake and drinking thick black coffee from chipped mugs. Before I was really conscious, I was dressed and eating the hunk of fresh baguette spread with butter and jam that constituted our free breakfast. We were all nervous but willing to show it in varying amounts, from the "I'm sure it will be nothing" bravado of the young Italian doctor who had started her walk to Santiago in Rome to the "Would it be so bad to just get a cab?" of a Canadian senior citizen. We left before the sun rose, a silent gaggle walking uphill, struggling with our heavy packs and worried minds.

The trail did not involve any sort of a warm-up period. It was unrelentingly steep from the beginning. As the sun topped the pine trees, I sweated, panted, and tried to just focus on putting one foot in front of the other. The happy exclamations of more fit pilgrims drew me to look up from my boots, and behind and below me I saw the village of Saint-Jean spread out like a storybook illustration. Tiny red roofs, white houses, green lawns, the castle seeming tiny from such a distance, its stone ramparts looking like a children's playset. If the perfection of Saint-Jean in miniature wasn't surreal enough, ahead of me an old man pulled to the side of the path and from his pack pulled a sort of bagpipe the size of a beach ball. He began to play the Irish anthem "Danny Boy." The instrument was made for mountains— the melody bounced across the rocks and vibrated in the trees before gliding down to the village below, a gentle rain of notes.

Was this real? Was such beauty even possible? With wonder I recalled my time in the hospital so many years before, when I had wanted to take my own life. How fortunate could one person be? To not only survive but to make it to this place, this music, these mountains? What a blessing to be alive at all, much less to be here. I spun in a complete circle, taking in the miracle of blue sky and green hills, of wandering melodies and the faces of pilgrims from nations near and far. Laughter bubbled out of me like a burbling fountain. Such joy, to walk through the valley of deepest depression and live to hear "Danny Boy" ring across sapphire crags.

In holy ecstasy, I laughed, delighted with the blessings raining down on me. I was alive in that moment. There was no past or future; I inhabited it fully. But a gentle-yet-purposeful cough from behind reminded me that a line of pilgrims on the trail below were waiting for me to begin walking again. I was blocking the narrow path. I trudged on, trying to keep the feeling of feather-light joy alive as my feet began to ache and my muscles strained.

Hours later, in a stupor from exhaustion, I walked above the tree line. From that height, the village disappeared. Below me, the great green blanket of forest was occasionally crossed by a tiny thread of a road or a brownish patch of clearing. All around was clean, thin air and cerulean mountains. Sheep, brought up to graze for the summer and early fall, stood in huge herds around the trail. Streaks of red, blue, or green spray paint across their backs denoted which farmer they belonged to. The sheep chewed methodically, uninterested in the constant stream of pilgrims cooing at them and taking their picture. Occasionally the whole flock would move from one area to another, some secret signal indicating that the grass was tastier on the other side of the trail. We humans would stop as they thundered in front of us, pointedly oblivious to we interlopers. Smaller herds of cows also grazed, and the bells around their necks rang out melodically in a seeming call and response from one group to another.

I stopped to sit on a large rock and eat an apple I had stowed in my pack. Although the sky was clear for hundreds of miles in every direction, the wind suddenly picked up, strong enough to send pebbles skittering off the ridge and make the sheep bleat in complaint. The cowbells rang more insistently, and the handkerchief covering my hair escaped, dancing down the mountain, a tie-dyed Camino escapee. I began to walk quickly, eyeing a tight ridge a few hundred yards ahead, a sort of high bridge with steep drops on either side. Anxiety filled first my stomach, then chest, then oozed into every limb as I considered that pass. The cows and sheep were beginning to meander to a lower altitude—should that be a sign? Could I be blown off the ridge, following my scarf over the cliffs onto sharp peaks below?

My anxiety disorder is familiar enough that when panic strikes, I realize it might be for illogical reasons. The solution is finding a reliable person to check in with, someone I trust to tell me if a situation is worth worrying about. On the Camino that task was harder—I didn't know anyone. I am not shy; I wasn't worried about talking to strangers. The problem was finding someone with my same sense of what was safe and what wasn't. I didn't want to ask an adrenaline-addicted base jumper if she was worried—some people don't worry enough. I wanted a person who worried a reasonable amount. Not a fretter like me, and definitely not a let's-swim-with-the-sharks type, but a sensible person.

The path was wide at this elevation, and it was easy for several people to walk abreast. I began to shop for my new sensible friend. I quickly disqualified the first pair I talked with, young Australians discussing ways to hammer camping hammocks into sheer rock face when climbing. Definitely not worrywarts enough for me. The next pair were South Korean. They had prepared for the Camino by learning quite a bit of Spanish. I had done the same, or so I thought until I actually started talking to Spanish speakers, who looked at me as if I was trying to communicate in Swahili. The South Koreans and I got past "How are you, where are you from," in Spanish but not any further. To save us all a lot of frustration, I smiled and moved on.

Meanwhile, I was getting closer and closer to the high ridge. Plenty of other pilgrims were moving across it, leaning steeply into the increasingly powerful wind but managing to stay on their feet. Still, the gales were getting stronger and stronger. Finally, I approached a retired schoolteacher from England. She had a no-nonsense haircut and sensible, well-broken-in hiking boots. She looked like the kind of person who could make a fire and a big pot of stew out of downed tree branches and a rabbit she caught with a trap made from the dental floss she always carried. Being English, she seemed surprised by my friendliness, but we started talking about the Camino route, and soon I felt sure that she was just the right amount of sensible to speak to about my fears.

KATE: Awful lot of wind.

ENGLISHWOMAN-WITH-SENSIBLE-HAIRCUT: Indeed. It's making the journey more difficult, though I'm not one to complain.

KATE: Yes, it's tiring walking against the wind. Do you think it will blow us off the ridge, dashing us across the rocks below, while in our agonizing pain our internal organs tumble across the valleys, to be eaten by the sheep and cows?

ENGLISHWOMAN: ... No. What? (*Annoyed*) I can never tell if Americans are kidding.

KATE: I'm just saying, it seems dangerous. The sheep and cows have moved down the mountain.

ENGLISHWOMAN: Don't say "I'm just saying," just say it. Do you really think you'll be blown off the mountain? With your pack, you are what, 200 pounds?

KATE: Well, a little less than that. ...

ENGLISHWOMAN: Americans and their safety regulations. You'd have to sign a thousand waivers before doing this at home, wouldn't you? You are fine, dear.

KATE: I wish there was a handrail to hang on to.

ENGLISHWOMAN: This is a mountain, not Disneyworld. No safety rails, but chin up, we'll make it.

We did indeed make it across, torsos bent to ninety degrees as we pushed against the wind. It took a long time to go the short distance, but when we got across the path took us to a lower altitude and out of the wind. Soon we were in the refuge of the trees, having crossed from Spain to France at some unmarked border, and I felt as light as a soap bubble without the resistance of the wind. Without the howling gale, the world was quiet. My thoughts returned to handrails of the spiritual sort.

In Unitarian Universalism, we seek holy wisdom in many faiths. Our spirits are free to roam as free as soap bubbles, landing on the practical living skills that come from the Buddhist Eight-Spoked Wheel, the Jewish inspiration of tikkun olam that moves us to heal the world, and great thinkers like Ralph Waldo Emerson who found divine unity in the woods of New England. We do not restrict our thought to one belief, one book, or one savior. Ninety percent of the time this freedom feels magnificent—I alight wherever my spirit encourages me. But once in a while it feels like walking across a high ridge without a handrail.

It's not the easiest religion to be a part of. Sometimes, when I feel afraid, when anxiety floods my body, I wish I believed in a God that was always looking out for me, who had a plan for my life. So even when everything was going wrong, I would know it was part of the plan. It would be nice to believe that I was on the true religious path, that I was in the correct church, doing the right rituals, guaranteed a happy afterlife. But mental illness introduced ambiguity to my life. All my absolutes crumbled under the crushing bulk of depression. Friendships, theology, even my own thoughts became unreliable. And as the depression dissolved, all that was left was mystery. Free thought. There was no turning back—the handrail was gone.

My Unitarian Universalist faith tradition comes from two older denominations, the Unitarians and (wait for it) the Universalists. Both were incarnated in the earliest version of the United States as a reaction to Puritanism, more specifically the philosophies that humans were born sinful and needed a good spiritual scrub-down on a regular basis and that without that scrub-down they would find themselves in Hell. Unitarians and Universalists questioned why God, who you may recall is in this Christian context supposed to be pretty awesome, would create humans just to damn them. Universalists added, "We see mothers with their children—toddlers who refuse to put on shoes, who won't eat anything that isn't beige—and yet the mothers manage to love these children. Even with all the toddlers' provocations, they love them. Shouldn't God be that good? The God that made us, that made patient parents, must be at least kind enough to forgive us our human errors."

In a weird, very human way, the Puritans were trying to add handrails to their terrifying existence in the New England colonies. Food was scarce; fires and disease ran rampant. They didn't know how to grow food in the harsh climate. They thought they were moving to a new, empty land to build a civilization—but Native Americans already occupied that land, already had governments and educational systems, behavioral norms and languages the Puritans didn't understand. They were scared and so they put handrails on their faith. They created structures to guarantee that while this life was quite a mess, if they followed the rules, they might get to have eternal happiness with God in the afterlife.

This is what we humans do: when we get scared, we try to add external handrails to our religious beliefs. As our climate catastrophe grows ever more apparent and dangerous, we hear from fundamentalist leaders that this is a test from God, that we need to live more moral lives to prove we don't deserve this punishment. So they kick their gay kids out of the house and keep women from accessing reproductive care, even though none of that is in the Bible. Church leaders make up new rules, rules that don't make any sense when looking at the whole picture of Christianity—a loving God, a gentle Jesus, and a never-ending Niagara Falls of forgiveness. Fundamentalists have weaponized their anxiety to create rules about how a Christian may or may not live and claim that this is the only way to prevent climate catastrophe. And they are right that many of the effects of climate change can be mitigated. We can be saved. But it will be by reducing carbon emissions and protecting the Amazon and funding alternative energy, not by kicking out gay kids. We need to pull together to save human existence, not make up rules about who is in and who is out based on fear.

Unitarians and Universalists didn't buy into the handrails the Puritans were building, and we don't buy what the fundamentalists are pushing now. We aren't a faith built on fear. Yes, this is a terrifying time to be alive. Humans have changed the ecosystems we live in to the point that we might not be able to live in them anymore. Whoops. But this is no time to make up random rules in order to please a God who doesn't exist. We won't worship a God who creates humans in order to damn them, whether with hell-fire or climate catastrophe.

Claiming that climate change is happening because God is angry and that we can mitigate that anger (and human extinction) by doing certain things, is lazy theology. Why would a loving God create us just to damn us? Better to think of ourselves as created in love in order to protect the magnificent gift that is our planet. It is scary to face a future that is so uncertain, but we will face it together. Not by creating fake handrails but by encouraging and comforting each other as we travel that path.

I made it through the wind and over the mountain not because of a bargain I made with an angry God but because a brisk-but-kind Englishwoman talked me through it. Walking in the quiet forest afterwards, I reflected that talking each other through the scary times is how Unitarians and Universalists survived the early days in the colonies and how we UUs will survive our current climate calamity. There will be holy ecstasy, the kind I experienced when the bagpiper played "Danny Boy" on our mountain ascent. And a lot of uncertainty, which comes when a religion's leaders respect people enough not to offer pat, lazy theology. We will make it through if we keep encouraging each other.

33.

But You'll Die!

It was Christmas Eve, and the church kids were strung out on sugar and the thrill of gifts to unwrap. Wearing footie pajamas and remnants of their Christmas pageant costumes, they swatted at their siblings with the shepherd's crooks. Angel halos toppled off into the water fountain as they slurped, sweaty and raucous. Parents were attempting to herd them into cars, grandparents were taking pictures, and I was thinking about getting home and into my own pajamas.

Sean, a kindergartner, came over for a final high-five on his way out the door, and I told him I liked his shirt. It was a cartoon man snowboarding. I wanted to try snowboarding, I told him. One of the big kids, a teenager at church, was teaching lessons at a nearby ski lodge and said he would teach me. I thought that sharing this information would make me seem cool, but Sean was appalled.

"No! No no no no NO!" he said. "You can't! You'll die!"

Sean's moms looked puzzled. "Reverend Kate can go snowboarding, hon. It isn't dangerous. You've tried it."

"No! She's so old. She'll die! I don't want her to die." Looking at me, clasping my hands as if begging me for mercy, he cried, "Please don't go. You are too old. You'll die."

Sean's poor parents. I couldn't stop laughing, he was upset, they were embarrassed. "You're not that old!" they kept saying, but to a five-year-old? I am ancient. At the time I was thirty-seven or so. Sean probably thought I rode a dinosaur to school when I was his age. But what I appreciated about the conversation was the love Sean was expressing. He didn't want me to die because I am important to him.

Ministers get a lot of feedback, to put it lightly. We hear about the pace of hymns and the lights being too low to read the hymn books, the sermon being to academic or too woo-woo, and what is with that tapestry the aesthetics team picked out? People mean well—their spiritual community is important to them, worship services are important to them, so they have strong feelings about things. Most days I remember that. But every once in a while, I want to yell, "I am doing my best here!" and then hide under my desk.

Spiritual community is where we get to practice being human together. Kiddos like Sean get to try out different ways of expressing affection, like telling their minister they are old, hearing adults laugh, and figuring out how it could go better. It's a safe place to make mistakes and try again.

Congregations are like laboratories for finding out which elements work together—a little humor, a lot of kindness—when moving in our people-filled world.

We practice relationships that are unlike any other—relationships that aren't transactional or based on family bonds, aren't organized toward meeting a goal or making a profit. In Unitarian Universalist congregations, we don't share a common theology but are experimenting with living according to certain values. What would it mean to remember that every person has inherent worth and dignity? That we are all tied in an interdependent web, with our choices impacting living creatures we may never encounter? How can we move toward a more just world, acknowledging the white supremacy interwoven in our culture? How do we face all the privileges we have benefited from?

In my denomination, we white folks are wrestling with the white privilege that has benefited us our whole lives. That benefited us before we were even born, when our ancestors were given land to farm or ranch on the western frontier, when white vets were given the GI Bill, when white folks were given great deals on federally insured home loans while Black folks faced redlining that kept them out of desirable neighborhoods. My parents got well-paying jobs in banks and department stores that didn't hire Black people. I went to a mostly white school that was better funded than the schools attended by mostly Black kids. I don't face the terrorism of police violence, and I am not afraid of being treated unfairly in the court system. I have loads and loads of privileges that I did not earn based on my melanin-challenged skin.

What does it mean to be in a faith community that proclaims "the inherent worth and dignity of every human" when Black people and people of color both inside and outside our doors face daily violence and discrimination? It means acknowledging that we live in a white supremacist culture that favors white people in every way. When I was a child, I thought white supremacy was a Ku Klux Klan member burning crosses on a Black family's lawn. Now I realize that white supremacy is threaded intricately in the tapestry of life in Western culture. It pops up everywhere: the bright red blood of Black children murdered by white police officers. The vivid orange of Black people in prison jumpsuits, victims of biased juries and "stop and frisk" policies. The hot pink of hair straightener smoothed into Black hair to make it look more like white hair, the burning chemical torture necessary to look "professional" in a world where looking professional equals looking white. The yellow of the news anchor's hair as she frets about welfare queens and the myth of the absent Black father.

It hurts in my chest and in the pit of my stomach when I think of the scourge of white supremacy. But because I am white, I can turn away from that pain, decide not to acknowledge it. This is another privilege. I can ignore Black suffering. For years and years, I have, choosing not to think about the fraternity on my college campus that was associated with the local Klan. Even when Black students expressed discomfort, I ignored them, choosing to be comfortable. When a Black friend told me that she hesitates to go to the protests that I frequent—legal, nonviolent marches and sit-ins— because of her fear of police retaliation. When I was in a shop with a Buddhist spiritual teacher and she grabbed a cart, declaring that even though she was only getting a few things, she couldn't carry them in her hands for fear of being accused of shoplifting.

It is infinitely more comfortable to ignore white supremacy culture. I can achieve "well-meaning white person" status by simply stating that racism and racists are bad. It is as easy as bemoaning the large-scale acts of violence against Black people by white people unashamed of being called racists. It is much more painful to see the racism in myself. It's much harder to acknowledge that all that I have accomplished is not due to my inherent awesomeness but because of white privilege. Plus, speaking up about the subtle racism in statements like "that's so ghetto" or "I'm just not into Black guys" makes my white friends and family uncomfortable. It causes them unease and might make me ostracized. Who wants to be the annoying one at the party?

The problem is that we all grew up, every one of us, with this idea that racism was this horrible, unforgivable sin and that it was committed by white men in white hoods burning crosses on people's lawns. Robin Di'Angelo speaks eloquently about this in her book *White Fragility*. We learned about racism as this cardinal sin that manifested in hate crimes, in apartheid, in slavery. Racism was the great evil and we were encouraged to remain vigilant, lest we become infected. And yes, racism does manifest in the KKK burning crosses, in slavery, in apartheid. But it also manifests in a billion small actions and inactions, like the city official who tried to save a few bucks by sending lead-dosed water to Flint, Michigan, which is predominantly Black. It manifests in a huge outcry from everyday white people when a Black woman is cast as Ariel in the upcoming remake of *The Little Mermaid*. These people don't think of themselves as racist, but they sure are mad about a kid's movie character having brown skin. Racism is embedded in our culture to the point where everyone is at least a little racist. I recall my brief jolt of surprise the first time I had a Black doctor—was it racist of me to be surprised? Sure. But I am kinda racist, just like just about everybody else in this world.

We were taught that racism was this horrible, evil force out there—but it is also the jolt of surprise at having a Black doctor. It's the everyday microaggressions, like hair products for Black women being in the ethnic section instead of under Haircare, which is products for white women. It is a white Seattle teacher reporting that she felt unsafe with a Black fifth grader—an adult afraid of a ten-year-old she is supposed to be teaching. Racism isn't "out there," it's everywhere. I know that nearly everyone is racist and that means me too. But we can do better. The first step is recognizing our own white supremacist thoughts and the racist structures that benefit us.

In our spiritual communities we get to practice what it means to be human, to be the best possible versions of ourselves. The best possible version of myself is learning to recognize white supremacy and my own racist notions. The best possible version of me is talking to other white people about racism because that is how we can dismantle it. It isn't fun or easy, but it is the only way we can get to a world where every person is treated like they have inherent worth and dignity.

When Sean told me that I was too old for snowboarding, he was saying the right thing—"I love you and don't want you to die"—in an awkward way. Fortunately, church is the perfect place to make this kind of mistake. In congregations we practice being our best self. They are great places for white people to learn from each other about white supremacy, to uncover our own racist assumptions, so we can do better when we are outside church walls. It isn't comfortable or fun or easy, but it is necessary if we are going to build the kind of world we dream about on Sunday mornings.

The year after Sean told me I was too old to snowboard, his family moved out of state. He made me a goodbye card with two airplanes drawn on the front. One airplane was larger and flying over the little airplane, shielding it. The big airplane was labeled Rev. Kate, and the little one was labeled Sean. Inside it said, "You rock like a jet plane." Love, perfectly communicated.

34.

Jazz Hands for the Prodigal Son

WHEN I WAS LITTLE, the children in my congregation put on a musical each year, a Biblical story with easy folk harmonies and lots of jazz hands–based choreography. I imagine they were pretty hard to watch, but the adults in the congregation praised us like we were headed for Broadway, and I have always loved any excuse to receive applause. Every year we pulled on glue-gun assembled costumes and sang about Adam's apple or Daniel in the lion's den. But the production I remember the best is the one about the Prodigal Son.

The Prodigal Son, for you heathens that grew up deprived of Bible stories transmitted via peppy song-and-dance performances, is in the book of Luke, in the New Testament. It's a parable, which means a made-up story that teaches a lesson. Some of the people hearing the story were Jewish, some were not, and the goal of the story was to convert people to Jesus' version of newly reformed Judaism. In the Prodigal Son parable, there are three characters, a dad and two sons. They are farmers, and well off enough that the boys are set to inherit land and wealth. Trouble is, the younger son is tired of the physical hardship of farm work. He is bored living out in the country. So he asks his dad for his inheritance and heads to the big city.

Once the country mouse is in the big city, he squanders his money on wild living. As a child I had no idea what wild living meant—nothing but ice cream sundaes for dinner? Staying up later than 9 PM? In our musical version, the prodigal son was played by Alice Walters, the most beautiful girl in church and perhaps in Dayton, who had blonde hair and huge green eyes and sang prettier than Debbie Gibson. Alice was always the lead in everything. She was even Adam in *Adam's Apple* (the director was very progressive in his casting choices. Also, Alice was the only one with any actual singing talent).

Alice was directed to act out the wild living of the prodigal son by pretending to buy lots of jewelry and eat lots of food and to buy food and jewelry for her friends too. Of course, as soon as the prodigal son's money ran out, his friends disappeared. He had to get a job feeding pigs, where he realized that the pigs were eating better than he was. Ouch. So he heads home, planning to hang his head in shame at losing his fortune and beg to be hired as a servant. He hopes to be given a bed among the pigs in the barn and maybe an old donkey blanket. It is more than he deserves, but he remembers that his father is a kind man.

From far, far away, his father sees his son approaching and runs to him, embracing him. He shouts for a celebratory feast to be prepared and for a fine robe to cover his son's shoulders. In my mind, I see the father weeping with joy, tears running into his mouth as he laughs, nearly hysterical with joy. I see a hug that lasts five minutes as the father breathes in the scent of his boy, the precious scent he has known since his son's birth.

I was thinking about the prodigal son recently while talking to a woman planning her dad's funeral. Her dad, Paul, was a long-time churchgoer, a gruff man with a soft heart and twinkly eyes. When I started at the church, seven years before, he told me he had a daughter who lived nearby and a son who had died in an accident when he was a teenager. The boy was returning the Christmas lights to the loft in the garage, and he became tangled in the cords and fell onto the cement floor. But that story wasn't true. That was the cover story, carefully woven to hide a deep, excruciating well of pain. The agony of the prodigal son's father, whose son didn't return.

Paul was away at sea most of the time when his children were growing up. He was a marine, and when the war ended, he stayed in the armed forces, having no high school diploma or other training. His wife had one child and then two, and he saw them a few times a year. Paul felt guilty about being away nearly all of the time, and when he was home, he believed he should be the disciplinarian his father had been, but even more exacting since he was around so little. Six months' worth of discipline in six days. His little girl learned to perfect her manners when he was around, the model of a well-behaved daughter. But her older brother rebelled. Paul and his son fought and fought and fought, miserable battles that ended in slammed doors and, on the worst day, in a fistfight.

Paul was away at sea, just off the coast of Brazil, when his superior officer sat him down and told him his son was dead. The boy hung himself in the garage while his mother and sister were running errands. Paul vomited, but he never cried. He didn't say a word. He packed a bag and caught a flight home. He and his wife arranged a small funeral, full of people who had been told the boy died in an accident. Only Paul's wife and daughter knew the truth. And they never talked about it—not one time. From the moment Paul walked in the door to the moment he returned, a week later, to the Marines, they never talked about it. Paul did not utter the name of his son to his daughter, not one time, until his wife died and he asked the cemetery if they could put her in a plot next to the boy's.

Paul's daughter spent her life attempting to stay the model of a well-behaved daughter. Despite her brother never being mentioned, she felt that he was constantly present, looming just out of sight. She was sure that her parents didn't mention him because they felt the wrong child had died. It was the 1960s and sons were prized. Her brother had gotten all of her dad's attention, even when that attention was negative. Now the prodigal son was gone, and if she was perfect, maybe her dad would pay attention her. So she became a scientist, because Paul loved science, and earned degree after degree, racked up honor after honor. And still he didn't seem to notice.

In the biblical parable, the prodigal son's brother has a difficult time accepting his brother's return. After all, he stayed on the farm. He has been tilling the fields and picking the olives while his brother partied in the city. He refuses to join the welcome-home party for his prodigal brother. His father pleads with him—it's like your brother died and came back to life! We thought we would never see him again, and here he is, with us!

When I was little, the story of the prodigal son was about forgiveness: no matter what you do, God will still love you. God will still welcome you home. The teller of the parable is talking to a diverse group of people—nonpracticing Jews, people from other religious groups, Jewish teachers and priests. And through the story he is saying, look—however you have worshipped God in the past, whether through elaborate rituals in the temple or sacrifices to nature deities or maybe just through trying to live an ethical life, God is super glad to see you whenever you show up. God's love is unconditional. So come on home—God is ready to throw a party in your honor.

My dream for congregations is that we can embody this parable. Let's be the prodigal son's father, running across the field to embrace all who seek community. Even if they have engaged in wild living, like ice cream sundaes for dinner. Even if they are broke and have been sleeping with the pigs. Even when they smell bad and are strung out. Even if they are an absent, hard-to-please father whose son committed suicide.

Paul's son didn't come home, and he thought his sin, his failure as a father, was unforgivable. Paul spent the rest of his life punishing himself. So his daughter labored without ceasing, trying to be successful enough to heal her father's heart. And so the trauma of the boy's death passed, unhealed, onto the next generation, who also dared not speak his name.

But, in my very best daydreams, Paul came to church the Sunday after his son died. And he ran into the arms of his spiritual community, and there he was embraced. In their loving arms, he told them the whole story: that he didn't know how to love his children other than to discipline them. That he feared his son's death was all his fault. That he couldn't imagine a day when he wouldn't berate himself. And his people, his congregation, would cover him with the healing balm of their own stories—parenting disasters and deep valleys of guilt and the excruciating agony of losing a child to suicide. And slowly he would heal. His wife and daughter, allowed to speak the boy's name, would heal. Not forget, but carry on, changed. Newly baptized into the pain of losing a child, newly washed in the grace of understanding that to be human is to fail, to forgive and be forgiven, and try again the next day.

We are all prodigal sons, children of many ages who have failed our parents, our loved ones, our own expectations of how we thought we would turn out. We all have fallen short of who we long to be. We are not as dependable or loving or successful or witty as we would like. Still, we yearn to run into loving arms. We ache to be enfolded in a spiritual community that recognizes that even in our brokenness we are holy. Can we be that community for each other? Can we enfold other people in the way we long to be enfolded?

When we recognize that even our own failures are forgivable, that even our worst sins don't keep us from being lovingly embraced by God, we can extend that grace to each person we meet. It isn't easy; remembering that we are lovable, or perhaps learning it for the first time, is difficult work. It is easier when we surround ourselves with people who love us. When I was a child, I was cherished by the adults at church, who helped me make glue-gun costumes and applauded my hammy performances in our musicals. Feeling cherished meant that even when I failed—which I did plenty—I never doubted that I could run home into their open arms. Even when I smelled like pigs and returned empty-handed, they wrapped me in a fine robe and called for a feast to be prepared in my honor.

Now that I am an adult, I extend the same unconditional love to the children and teenagers in my congregation. I weep with delight every time I fear that they are lost and then see them across the field, walking toward me. Overjoyed that they are returning home.

Benediction

Most Sundays, the church service wraps up with a benediction, a fancy church word for a couple of sentences the minister says before everyone can descend on coffee hour like a swarm of locusts who have never had cookies before. It is a quick wrap-up of the service plus a pep talk. If you had to write a benediction for this book, dear reader, what would it say? We have shared stories both funny and sad; we traveled over intense emotional terrain. Now what?

I want you to know that you are loved beyond your wildest imaginings by the spirit of creation. Every bit of you is holy—even the embarrassing parts, even the thoughts you wouldn't tell your best friend. God is in your every cell, calling you to live a loving, joyful, boisterous life. To go easier on yourself. To accept that you are a blessing. To spread the word that there is no original sin, that we are all glorious gifts to a world that desperately needs us.

I want you to know that you are a strand in the web of all existence, one dewdrop-spangled thread reflecting the early morning sun. Connected to every other living creature. Frogs, mushrooms, great blue whales, and you. You are never alone. You were born into a huge family of life. Sit in the grass and know that it is your sibling. Watch the crows circle and think of them as gossiping cousins. This is your world and you are worthy.

I used to worry a lot about doing religion right. If I got baptized and didn't have sex and loved my neighbor, then I could get into heaven, right? Right? But I wasn't really looking for God. I just wanted fire insurance—some guarantee that I wouldn't go to Hell. However, the more I searched for God, the more I pondered holiness, the less I believed in Hell. The more I believed that love was the nature of our being, I stopped looking for salvation and started thinking about how to live a meaningful life. A holy life. And around every bend I found real salvation—a connection with a spiritual community, the realization that I was a sacred being, that I wasn't broken but am deeply beloved.

The ancients told stories and wrote parables to explain what they had found when exploring the mystery. That is all religion is: people wondering about where we came from, why we are here, and where we go after we die. The Bible, the Eightfold Path of Buddhism, the Seven Principles of my own Unitarian Universalist tradition—all are just ideas people had about what made life meaningful. What you think about holiness is just as valid and just as true. So what *do* you think about holiness? What do you think about God? There is nothing to be afraid of. Your spiritual quest begins now.